A Yorkshire Vet: The Next Chapter

A Yorkshire Vet:
The Next Chapter

Julian Norton

CORONET

First published in Great Britain in 2020 by Coronet
An Imprint of Hodder & Stoughton
An Hachette UK company

This paperback edition published in 2020

1

A CIP catalogue record for this title is available from the British Library

Paperback ISBN 9781529378375
eBook ISBN 9781529378351

Typeset in Electra LH by Palimpsest Book Production Ltd, Falkirk,
Stirlingshire

Printed and bound in Great Britain by Clays Ltd, Elcograf S.p.A.

Hodder & Stoughton policy is to use papers that are natural, renewable and
recyclable products and made from wood grown in sustainable forests.
The logging and manufacturing processes are expected to conform to the
environmental regulations of the country of origin.

Hodder & Stoughton Ltd
Carmelite House
50 Victoria Embankment
London EC4Y 0DZ

www.hodder.co.uk

To all those who continue the Herriot ethos.
And to Derek, the elderly cat.

If you can bear to hear the truth you've spoken
Twisted by knaves to make a trap for fools,
Or watch the things you gave your life to, broken,
And stoop and build 'em up with worn-out tools

'If', Rudyard Kipling

1. Adrenalin, Cortisol and Gin

There is a wooden sign at the top of Sutton Bank, directing visitors to 'The Finest View in England'. It is a spectacular view, stretching away over the Vale of York to the Yorkshire Dales in the distance. It was the favourite view of famous vet James Herriot, and it was he who gave it its title. My favourite view, however, was a little less breathtaking. It was the view from my consulting room window, across our car park, towards some industrial and commercial buildings on the other side of the road. My first job on arrival at the practice, every working day for almost twenty years, was to open the blinds, allowing the sunlight to flood in and me to see out.

I liked the view because I could see all the cars approaching, carrying worried owners with sick pets, and Land Rovers with farmers collecting medicines or wanting to chat about a cow with mastitis or lambing problems. I could recognise the vehicle of a particular farmer or cat-owner, giving me advance warning of what I might be required to do. During a busy afternoon or evening surgery, as I drew up a vaccine or tidied up between consultations, I could watch my patients making their way to the front door.

As Rufus the elderly Sheltie hobbled across the car park, I could peer out and observe how he was managing with that painful left hock. The stubborn old boy defied all expectation, as he collected every medical and surgical condition known to veterinary medicine, but I worried about him. From my window, I could see how fast he walked, or if his owners needed to carry him – surely a bad sign.

I watched as Winston, the stout and stoic bulldog, cocked his leg on a conifer tree. The length of time it took him to empty his bladder showed me how well his bladder condition was progressing. Observation is a vital part of making a diagnosis or monitoring a condition, and my window gave me the perfect opportunity to do this, catching my patients relaxed and off guard before the anxieties of a trip to the vet set in.

Sometimes a horsebox would appear, obstructing the entrance, and the next free vet would head out to treat the horse in the car park. In spring, that same car park could become a makeshift maternity ward as farmers arrived with ewes to lamb. It saved us a trip to the farm, and saved the farmer a bit of money, but not everyone in the practice was so keen: 'It just makes such a mess in the car park,' lamented one of my colleagues. 'All that blood and straw and mess! We should get them to shovel it back into their trailer and take it back to the farm!'

But, at the end of afternoon surgery on a gloomy Wednesday in March of 2017, it was not the prospect of a difficult lambing that caused me concern. It was the purposeful striding of two large gentlemen towards the front door of Skeldale that made my heartbeat quicken and my stomach lurch. I had not seen them before, but I knew who they were and I knew their intentions. I also knew that their arrival signalled the beginning of some big and unwanted challenges.

I'd experienced this panicky sensation before, but only in extreme circumstances; the time when, in 1995, a car clipped the back wheel of my mountain bike during an ill-timed manoeuvre across an otherwise quiet country road, sending me flying through the air and, luckily for me, into the hedge; the time I returned to my car, which I had left outside Tesco, only to discover that my four-year-old son wasn't sitting in the car seat where I had left him. I had rushed in to buy spaghetti to feed some unexpected visitors. I told him I would be back by the time he had counted to one hundred. I knew I could do it in time. But he had got to one hundred more quickly than I had expected and he needed a wee, so he had taken himself to the toilet in the supermarket. He was fine (and continued to wander off on a reasonably regular basis for years to come), but my adrenal glands had been well and truly squeezed.

I also experienced this feeling at six o' clock one Thursday morning in the summer of 2001. The country was in the grip of the foot-and-mouth disease epidemic and I was at the Thirsk Auction Mart, checking cattle and sheep for signs of the disease before they were loaded onto wagons to be moved. My phone rang. It was a farmer calling about his heifers. They were all standing still in the field, salivating profusely. These were the signs of foot-and-mouth disease. It was a moment of veterinary catastrophe.

Now, as I watched the two portly gentleman approach, I had the feeling that this could be another veterinary catastrophe.

I finished with my last patient and they appeared at my consulting room door.

'We're from the dark side,' one of the men joked as they introduced themselves, each thrusting out a hand for me to shake.

They had already had a meeting with my partners, over lunch in a local hotel. I had not attended. I couldn't attend. It was a busy day and I had been out pregnancy-testing some cows for a farmer who had a small herd of Dairy Shorthorns. Martin's cows meant the world to him, but his small enterprise was more of a hobby than a livelihood, so visits had to be arranged to fit around his other job – the one that paid his bills. Late on a Wednesday morning was the only time he could get away from his respon- sibilities on the pig farm where he worked, so the clash was unavoidable. When it came to a choice between a meeting with representatives of the corporate side of veterinary practice, or my friend who needed his cows to be checked, there was only ever going to be one winner.

All Martin's cows were in calf. He was delighted. It meant that his chances of having an animal ready for the important summer shows looked hopeful. As I gathered up my kit and cleaned my wellies, I picked up a voicemail on my phone from the surgery, regarding a calf I had seen the previous day. The farmer was worried. The calf, who had severe scour, was still very weak. Bad diarrhoea can be fatal to a newborn suckler calf, so it would need some more vigorous treatment, as a matter of urgency. I said goodbye to Martin and headed over the moors to Old Byland to see what I could do.

By the time I got back, afternoon surgery had started. There was no time for lunch. As I had suspected, my partners were still in their meeting, bartering with the future of our practice, so the waiting room was full and the remaining vets were stretched.

But now I found myself shaking hands with two men claiming to be 'from the dark side'. I had a sick feeling in my stomach that had nothing to do with being up close and personal with a week-old calf with enteritis, and everything to do with the realisation that the shape of my future was being wrenched out of my hands. These two men would have their work cut out to persuade me that their intentions were good. I had made it very clear that I was not a fan of this type of practice. I was about as amused (to continue the *Star Wars* analogy) as Luke Skywalker would have been with such an introduction.

They wanted to buy the practice. They owned a large chain of veterinary practices, all small-animal clinics. They had both been veterinary surgeons themselves before branching out into acquisitions, and, in the discussion that followed, they related anecdotes of poorly dogs and injured cats in a bid to convince me that they were, in fact, 'one of us'. I did not need persuading of their provenance. I could tell it was many years since they had covered a night on duty, treated a calf with diarrhoea or even finished off a busy afternoon surgery. Their days were full of a different type of work. Their job was to persuade practice owners to sell them their veterinary businesses. I was not sure this was such a good idea.

I had spent more time at Skeldale than any other place in my entire life. Twenty-one years doesn't sound so long, but if you consider that working days started at 8.30 in the morning and finished at 7.30 in the evening if I was lucky, or midnight if I wasn't, and then add in the weekends that I have been on duty, the times I have dropped in to check on inpatients, sort out computer glitches on a Sunday evening or put out medication for clients and friends who've knocked on my door or sent me text messages about a sick pet, it amounts to a lot of time to spend in one place. This practice, the business of which I was a part, was not just my job; it defined me as a professional and was part of the very stuff that made me the person I was. And now this was threatened. My adrenal glands were in for some sustained work.

But, for the moment, there were still calls to be done. March is a busy time for veterinary surgeons in mixed practice. Today was no exception, and I had another sick calf to visit. However, the guests had a train to catch and it was, apparently, my job to take them to the station. As they climbed into my messy car, which smelt strongly of farm, I had a feeling that, despite their assertions that they were veterinary surgeons through and through, my new acquaintances would not be particularly interested in coming with me to see a calf belonging to an octogenarian farmer and his wife. That sort of work would certainly not fit into their business model. And I didn't want them to miss their train back to London. Thirsk railway station is positioned a mile and a half out of the town centre. This is inconvenient for visitors to the town and it was an inconvenience for me on this Wednesday afternoon.

If you look at a map of North Yorkshire, you can see how the north-eastern mainline makes a slight westward deviation around Thirsk, before heading north-east again on its route from York, via Northallerton towards Scotland. The story goes that, back in the days when railways were taking over from canals as the principal means of transporting goods around the country, the landowners of Thirsk were particularly suspicious of trains. *They* didn't want a newfangled machine, rolling along great metal girders, cutting through their land, nor did they want a whole load of new visitors spoiling their grazing and their town. If Thirsk *had* to have a railway station, it had to be 'out of town'. Had circumstances been different, and the station built near the centre of Thirsk, the small market town would surely have developed into something much bigger. Instead Northallerton, eight miles or so to the north, with its more centrally placed station, assumed the role of administrative centre for North Yorkshire and grew accordingly, with a hospital, a prison and even a department store! As I took my guests to meet their connection back to London, I silently berated those farmers from years ago for being so belligerent; it might have been a shorter and less uncomfortable drive.

Their parting words – 'Don't worry, Julian. It will all be fine.' – did little to help my soaring blood pressure. Nor did they ease my concern for the future. My plan had always been to continue the Herriot tradition at Skeldale, encouraging younger assistants to stay in the practice by giving them the chance to buy into the business, allowing both it and them to develop and move forward. To my mind, if the vet attending to a sick sheep during a long, dark January night feels they are an integral part of both the practice and the rural community, the business runs better and everyone is happier in their work. I had always been led to believe that, one day, I would have the chance to be the senior partner, and I had spent the last eighteen years working towards this point. In this new scenario, it seemed that neither I nor my younger colleagues stood any chance against the deep, venture-capital-backed wallets of investment-company-owned multiples. I felt deeply sad as the two large gentlemen made their way from my car to the steps of the station. I imagined they were delighted that they had sent out the first tendrils to net another acquisition. Although there would be much to discuss over the coming months, deep down I knew my life would never be the same again.

Veterinary practice has a good knack of smoothing out the low points with well-timed, happy moments. Only last week, the devastation of the dog on the operating table with an inoperable splenic tumour had soon evaporated as a litter of happy, healthy, squeaking cocker spaniel pups were delivered by emergency

Caesarean section. And luckily, on this day, my very next patient was the perfect antidote to my anxiety. I had an appointment with Mr and Mrs Green.

The case was spelt out clearly enough in the daybook. 'Green, Stoneybrough Farm. Calf pneumonia, ASAP.' On a damp and chilly afternoon in March, pneumonia is a common problem in the Vale of York, where mist hangs low for most of the day. The delicate lungs of little calves are particularly vulnerable, especially those calves from dairy farms, where they leave their mothers soon after they are born to be reared on milk replacer and tasty solid food. It is a system that works well on the whole, and there are many rearing units around this part of North Yorkshire. In years gone by, Stoneybrough Farm had its own dairy herd of about forty cows, all fastened by their necks in an old-fashioned cow byre. Everything about this farm was old-fashioned, including its owners, Steve and Jeanie Green.

I met Steve and Jeanie almost twenty-one years ago, soon after I started work in Thirsk. Theirs was one of the first farms I visited. I lived just over the road from Stoneybrough Farm, so a cow with milk fever would be a common early-morning job for me, on my way into the surgery, while a call in the evening to scouring calves or a cow to cleanse I could do on my way home. I had come to know the elderly farmers, their stock and their numerous cats and dogs very well.

'It's Treacle and Sponge,' bellowed Jeanie as I pulled up outside the farm. She wasn't referring to what was on the menu for pudding, but the sick calves – two, as it turned out, rather than just one. All the cattle on this farm had names, a tradition dating back to when the Greens kept milking cows. 'Buttercup', 'Daisy', 'Clover', 'Twinkletoes' and 'Sally' would all know their place in the cow byre. It was a sad day, in the summer of 2015, when the decision was made to sell the cows. A combination of advancing years, ill health and the rising challenges within the dairy industry, which made it almost impossible for a small dairy herd to function, all conspired to bring about an emotional end of an era.

Now, Steve and Jeanie's farming enterprise consisted of buying young calves in pairs, and rearing them to the size of 'store cattle' to be sold at Thirsk Auction Mart. This made a bit of money for the couple, but it was more about continuing a way of life than swelling the coffers of a rudimentary pension. For farmers, old habits die hard. Jean continued the tradition of naming her animals, and used names that worked well in pairs – Peaches and Cream, Rhubarb and Custard and so on. It put added pressure on the vet when treating a potentially life-threatening illness, because if the worst happened it was even more tragic to have just Peaches with no Cream. A similar thing often happens with kittens. People acquire two kittens together, so that they can keep one another company, and the obvious thing to do is to name them Gin and Tonic or Bubble and Squeak. This fills the vet with dread, that one will succumb to premature illness or have an early life calamity, leaving a single lonely kitten, forever missing half of its name.

But Treacle and Sponge were in safe hands with Steve and Jeanie. I donned my wellies and waterproof trousers and climbed over the gate into the farmyard, taking great care to stay at the hinge end so as not to put extra strain on the ancient metalwork. This was an important first piece of advice from wise and experienced farmers at Stoneybrough to a young and inexperienced vet. Standing on the wrong end of a gate, where the weight of a person puts more strain on its hinges, only serves to shorten the life of a farm gate. Everything on a farm is designed to last a lifetime – barns, sheds, tractors and farmers – and nobody wanted to add extra and unnecessary problems.

'How are they doing, Jeanie?' I asked as we made our way to

the calf shed. I needed to find out as much as I could – how long had the calves been on the farm, were they still on milk or had they started on calf pellets, were they eating or drinking? With as much information as I could gather before I actually set about my examination, I could make a better assessment of the two patients.

Both Steve and Jeanie came to help me manhandle the calves into a corner of the spacious, straw-filled pen in which they were living. The wooden hay manger, above a deep stone feed trough from a bygone era, was still full. Either they had been over-optimistic with how much a pair of young calves would eat, or the two Hereford crosses had gone off their food. Treacle was easily caught and I plugged my stethoscope into my ears to assess his lungs. There was the telltale rasp of a respiratory infection, extending throughout most of the little calf's chest. He sounded bad and Jeanie was right to be concerned. The next step was to check his temperature. There was a tradition at Stoneybrough whereby we all had to guess what the reading would be. Steve would always be conservative in his estimate: 'A hundred and three, I think. M'be hundred and three and a half,' he pondered.

'No Steve. It's way more than that!' exclaimed Jeanie. 'Look at his lugs – hanging down like that. If his lugs are down it's sure to be higher. I'd say Treacle's temperature is a hundred and five!' She was so certain, there was almost no need for my thermometer.

Sure enough, the mercury rose and kept rising and when it eventually stopped, I pulled the thermometer out and peered at the reading, before showing it to Jeanie. She was right.

'I told you so Steve – it's just shy of a hundred and five!' she exclaimed before doing a little dance around the calf-pen in celebration, before quickly regaining composure as she realised the gravity of the situation.

I moved on to Sponge, whose lugs were not so low and who was not so easy to catch. He skipped around the pen and was evidently not as poorly as his mate. But the stethoscope told a similar story – rattling and harsh noises. What would the temperature be? A hundred and three was the consensus and that's what it was. He was sick, but not quite so sick.

I gathered some medication from my car boot and injected both calves with antibiotics and anti-inflammatories, promising to return the next day to check on their progress. It wasn't quite a matter of life and death, but I knew everyone would feel happier to know things were proceeding in the right direction. In any case, they both needed another injection and I thought it would be much easier for me to do, rather than to leave the old couple to do battle with a needle and syringe as well as the unruly calves.

Steve and Jeanie were not your usual type of farm client. And Stoneybrough was not your usual type of farm. As if to emphasise the point, Jeanie shuffled off into the farmhouse and returned with an enormous bar of chocolate.

'There you go, lad,' she said as she thrust the family-sized bar into my hand. 'You look like you need it.' Jeanie was a kind lady.

I waved goodbye from the open window of my car. I would have liked to have stayed to chat for longer. After my unsettling afternoon meeting, it was nice to be doing what I loved, with old friends. However, evening surgery beckoned, it was already dusk and I was late. I knew the car park would be full again and there would be a queue of dogs and cats waiting for my attention. At least I had Jeanie's chocolate to keep me going.

An hour or so later, everyone who needed to be seen had been seen and I could finally head for home. It had been a hard day but at least it wasn't my night to be on duty.

'Have you had a good day?' asked Anne, my wife, with a

careful smile. A veterinary surgeon herself, she knew all about the ups and downs of general practice and she was used to my weary appearance at the back door at unpredictable times of night. I kicked off my shoes on the doormat.

'Well, it's been mixed,' I replied, although this seemed something of an understatement.

'All Martin's cows are pregnant, which is good. He's delighted and they are all set for calving at just the right time for the Great Yorkshire Show. He thinks he has a good chance of a prize this year. Mind you, he always thinks that!'

Anne nodded – Martin's Great Yorkshire Show dramas were an annual event.

'My calf with diarrhoea in Old Byland isn't much better,' I continued. 'I think it has salmonella [grimace from Anne], so that's not so good. I'm going back tomorrow to check it. Steve and Jeanie have an outbreak of pneumonia. Oh, and I met two blokes who said that they were from "the dark side". But it's probably going to be okay, because they said everything is going to be fine. So, a funny old day, really.'

I slumped into the nearest chair and felt my adrenal glands ache.

'Have we got any gin?'

2. Squaring the Circle

Despite the gin, I didn't sleep well that night. It was not the sick calves at Stoneybrough preying on my mind, nor was it the spectre of salmonella in Old Byland. It was the two men claiming to be from the dark side that kept me awake, and everything that their visit implied for the future of Skeldale.

During the small hours, I played through in my mind what might happen over the next few months. I'd already done some research and knew that their company owned several hundred small-animal practices. My investigations also told me that they had borrowed heavily, from both banks and venture capital companies, to fuel a shopping spree that would expand the company massively. They were clearly heading out of their southern heartland and reaching northwards. It sounded, and felt, like a medieval conquest. Our practice wasn't like any they had bought before. For a start, we were a mixed practice, dealing with farm animals and horses as well as pets. But we had a high profile. Not only was the practice probably the most historic veterinary surgery in the country, home as it had been to James

Herriot, but we were now on TV. They had us firmly in their sights. The fact that these gentlemen had appeared at the practice the previous afternoon, and that I'd been manoeuvred into taking them on a fifteen-minute car journey to the station to be persuaded of their good intentions, meant that my partners were actually thinking of selling it to them. Everyone knew that this was not a path I was interested in following. Until yesterday, I had thought I was not alone.

It was true that running a small, mixed, independent practice could be hard. The job was getting more difficult and the responsibility was certainly getting more challenging. It was also true that corporate takeovers were running apace through the profession. Even some 'die-hard' independent practices had recently gone corporate, 'selling out', literally and metaphorically. It is called 'consolidation of a fragmented industry'. The same process had occurred in pharmacies in the 1990s, and opticians, solicitors and dentists all followed a similar pattern in the 2000s. My mother had been a pharmacist at that time, working in several small, independently owned stores. The patients, who visited to collect their regular, life-preserving prescriptions – or 'scripts, as I knew them, from my mum's tea-time accounts of her day's work ('I did over three hundred 'scripts today,' she'd recall) – were as much friends as they were customers, and she would often drop off an oxygen cylinder to a housebound patient on her way home or offer reassurance and support when things got tough. Most of those local pharmacies were swept up in a wave of corporate buying, and their place at the heart of the community was often lost. The term 'fragmented industry' suggests there is something wrong – that the industry is somehow broken and that providing a good service to those in your community isn't enough. But, in my opinion, the veterinary profession wasn't broken. Or, at least, it wasn't until the corporates decided it needed to be consolidated.

To some the process was a good thing. The outgoing partners got an overinflated price for their business, while the investors got to apply economies of scale, extracting their return by improving efficiency: by using a single accountancy firm, for example – although, of course, this would be a national one, so the local firm, who had built a relationship with the practice over many years, would lose the work; by streamlining the supply process, using their enormous purchasing power to buy drugs more cheaply; by trimming the workforce and making those who remained work just that bit more efficiently (for that read work harder, for longer); by increasing the prices, calculating that the extra revenue would outweigh the relatively minor loss of clients – those clients who twigged what was going on, that is. Other clients would stay, through either loyalty or inertia, in the same way that you never get around to changing your bank or your energy supplier. The plan would be to double the profits of the practices that had been acquired, and then sell on to another equity powerhouse who owned even more veterinary practices, maybe even merging with a continental enterprise or one across the pond in the USA. (At the time of writing, an investment group based in continental Europe owns one major chain of UK veterinary surgeries, another is owned by shareholders and listed on the London Stock Exchange and a third is owned by the American giant, Mars. As in Mars Bars.) The pattern was a clear one and it certainly did not follow the Herriot tradition that I was keen to continue.

It's not that I'm against corporate-style practices. Much of what they can offer is very positive, provided it is done properly: a structured education programme, a proper HR department to support veterinary staff and the sharing of facilities and expertise between practices within the corporation for example; but it all seemed a million miles from what I'd been doing at Stoneybrough Farm that afternoon after my trip to the station, and it was not a circle I could square. At least not one I could square between the grim small hours of two and six in the morning. From whichever direction I looked, it didn't feel right for me, or for Skeldale, for many reasons.

So, the slightly nauseous feeling in my stomach over breakfast was a combination of lack of sleep and a deep anxiety for the future of the practice, and the future for my family and me. Whatever would transpire over the coming months, I knew there would be stress, difficult decisions and undoubtedly some major changes. I needed to find a way of squaring that circle and it would take more than one sleepless night. My first job was to investigate the company in more detail – or, in my *Star Wars* analogy, investigate the 'Empire' – although today my first job (after taking the kids to school) was actually to check up on Jeanie's pneumonic calves.

'How are they today, Jean?' I asked as I pulled into the yard.

'Treacle and Sponge are much better, thank yer very much,' declared Jeanie, ushering me into the shed with a flourish. Even before I had reached for my stethoscope and thermometer, I could see that the two little Hereford-cross calves were feeling much better. They had taken some milk for breakfast, Jeanie reported, and were now nibbling on the hay that yesterday was spilling, untouched, out of the manger. The calves were quite young to be eating much in the way of roughage, but even nibbling a mouthful or so was a good thing for the developing rumen, as the diet gradually shifted from mother's milk to herbage. At this farm, though, the calves would be given milk for an extended period. Every creature at Stoneybrough was treated like royalty. For a few years after the dairy company deemed it uneconomical to collect milk from their dairy farm, Steve and Jean continued to milk their cows, filling the small, stainless steel tank in the dairy next to the cow byre and then taking it in buckets to feed to the young cattle in the next-door shed. It was laborious work, but work that benefited the calves and resulted in sturdy young stock with shiny and glossy coats.

I was glad I had called in. Archie, my youngest son and a budding vet, went to school just up the road from the farm, so it was no trouble to call on my way past without having to charge for a visit. The calves' temperatures were normal and their lungs sounded better. It was a good start to the day, but as I headed to the practice, I knew I needed to find time to speak with my senior colleagues about the meeting. I needed to find out what they had been promised to make them even begin to consider this dramatic move.

By a quarter to nine I was in the office at the surgery, perusing the daybook and the ops list, working out a plan for the day and making a few phone calls. I wanted to check on my scouring calf again, but there was another, more pressing visit: a cow calving at one of my favourite farms. It was some distance away from the practice, to the north. I couldn't hang around, so I put my initials next to it, before adding a second note: '*JN – Manor Farm, Old Byland: Revisit scouring calves*'. That would be enough to keep me out of the surgery for most of the morning. I grabbed the Caesarean box, with the calving jack perched precariously on top, and headed out of the back door to my car.

The twenty-minute drive north to John's farm gave me more time to think about the future. This would be one of the last cows to calve this spring for John and his family. They had a fantastic herd, comprising some of the country's finest South Devon cattle. They were all superb specimens and the rich conker-brown of their coats told a tale of wonderful health and tip-top management. This was one of the first farms with which I became involved when I started work in Thirsk and I'd developed a strong bond with John, his son Jack and their various stockmen over the years. The calving pattern was tight and the herd was well organised. Four months ago, on a visit that always signified the onset of winter, I had pregnancy-tested all the cows in the herd, so we knew that there would be no calves born after the end of March. The bulls had left the cows by the end of June and, since the gestation period for a cow is nine months, today's calving was likely to be one of their last until next year. As I drove northwards, with the Hambleton Hills, which mark the edge of the Vale of York and the start of the North York Moors, rising up to the east, I considered that this might actually be the last calf I would *ever* deliver on this farm. If the men from the dark side had their way, it was unlikely I would still be in the practice when John's next calving period came round, and I doubted that the potential new owners would have much desire to continue to support our local farmers either, such was their obvious focus on small-animal work.

'Morning, Jack,' I called out of my car window as I rolled up outside the cowshed. 'Have we got some problems?'

'Morning Julian,' Jack called back as he came out to meet me. 'Thanks for coming. Yes, we have got problems. Dad's done it again. He's gone on holiday and left me in charge. We've only got two more cows to calve. I said I'd be okay to take charge for the last few – they're both old cows and I thought they'd calve by themselves. But this one's having trouble. The head's back and I just can't get it.'

I pulled on my wellies and headed for the hot water tap. I'd done this a hundred times before. I knew the water heater would be on and would give me just enough hot water to fill a bucket.

By the time I'd finished, unless the job was very quick, the water would be hot again, ready for me to clean up.

Warm water, lubricant, calving ropes and wooden sticks at the ready, I rolled up my sleeves for an initial feel. Jack was right. There were two feet but no nose. A calf with its head back can present a challenge. Firstly, the capacious size of a South Devon's abdomen can make it physically very difficult to even reach the head, let alone manipulate it into the correct position. Secondly, the reason that a head is back is often because there isn't sufficient space in the cow's pelvis for the front legs *and* the head. It can be an indicator of a tight problem. I would soon find out. I took off my shirt, to keep its rolled-up sleeves clean and allow me a few extra inches of reach, cleaned my arm and applied some lubricant. It was cold on this damp March morning.

'Your dad's done this before, hasn't he?' I asked, remembering a time when I'd been called out to a heifer, who was drooling profusely from her mouth and looking sickly. Jack had been in charge on that occasion too and had been filled with fear, certain that it was the return of the dreaded foot-and-mouth disease. Luckily, it wasn't anything of the sort. The unfortunate heifer had been chewing on a blackthorn bush and a huge, spiky piece of stick was lodged across the back of her mouth. With some difficulty, and with Jack's help to restrain her head, I had managed to remove the offending object, which immediately relieved her discomfort. She celebrated by escaping from her halter and careering off down the drive. I've never seen a farmer run so quickly, as Jack raced to reach the farm gate before the heifer. It was a close call, but he managed to close the open gate in the nick of time and disaster was averted.

We recounted the story together now, laughing about the successful outcome and what could have been disaster if the heifer had reached the open gate before Jack.

Then I stretched as far as I could to try to reach the calf. With some difficulty, I managed to hook a finger around the end of its nose and straighten the head. I was making progress, and tried to reassure Jack. I always feel sorry for a farmer in this situation. He is anxious about his cow and its unborn calf and, unless I provide a running commentary about what I can feel, he hasn't got a clue what the outcome might be. A huffing and puffing vet offers little reassurance, so I always try to explain what I'm doing. As soon as I lube my other arm, to use both hands, the farmer can start to feel more confident, because it means the head is up and the calf is coming. The only issue then is whether there is enough space. Today, I felt confident that this old cow would deliver her calf without any problems once the head was lined up and I asked Jack to pass the bucket containing my calving ropes.

'I think we're gonna be okay, Jack,' I reassured the young farmer. The calf's head was now in place, following behind the two front feet. They weren't too large and I was as sure as I could be that we'd be able to pull it out without too much trouble.

It was bigger than I expected, and the calf – a lovely chestnut-brown heifer – landed with a satisfying thud on the deep straw behind its mum.

'That's a good job, well done Julian. And thank you. Dad will be pleased,' said Jack. He was matter of fact but delighted at the same time.

I cleaned the bloody slime from my arms and washed my hands, before returning to watch mum and baby establish the bond that would last a lifetime. For me, this was the best bit of my job. Even on a busy day, or in the middle of the night in the depths of winter, I always spend a few minutes watching a young calf struggle to its feet, searching for a teat while mum's natural instincts to clean and dry the new calf kick in. It is nature at its best. In a sometimes difficult world, watching this handsome mum and her healthy baby bond was a special thing to be part of and I didn't want to leave. This mixture of emotions, along with the satisfaction of having been part of this birth and the obvious relief of the farmer, was a powerful drug and a habit I didn't want to kick.

I took the long route from Osmotherley to Old Byland. Well, it was actually the shortest route, but it wound up and over the hills so it was slower than taking the main road. Spring was still some way off in North Yorkshire, but there was already the hint of abundant new growth in the fields and there was definitely new life in the cowsheds. I climbed out of the village and across the open moors, where the roads did not have walls or hedges to prevent sheep from wandering across them. Up then down, round switchback bends and blind corners and then through the sleepy village of Hawnby, across a ford and up another steep hill and I would soon be back to see my poorly calf.

So far, it had been a good morning. My first two patients were better, the calving had been a success – a relief for cow, farmer and vet – and the drive across the moors was similarly cathartic. I resolved to put the traumatic events of yesterday and the anxious question mark over the future of the practice to the back of my mind. I would research the group who were intent on buying Skeldale to the best of my ability; I would try to do the best for my clients and for the practice, upholding its heritage, its tradition and its values as much as I could. I would argue my case and I would stand by my principles. As junior partner, if it came to a vote I was actually pretty impotent, but I resolved to do the right thing, whatever that turned out to be. I also resolved not to let it get me down and to stay positive. And with that in my mind, I arrived at the farm in Old Byland, hoping the little calf would have shown some improvement. I grabbed my stethoscope and thermometer and headed into the barn to see my patient. This was what I did best.

3. Unusual Jobs in March

March is a particularly busy time for a veterinary surgeon in mixed practice. Farm animals are still housed, which brings various problems not seen when they are outside in the sunshine, eating grass. It is also easier to do the routine veterinary jobs when cattle are inside, as they are all in one place and more straightforward to handle than they are when they have big fields to charge around. This is also the month when calving is in full swing and so is lambing. Days and nights are unpredictable and fun in equal measure.

However, the emergency I was called to on this particular March day was different from the usual March emergency. My patient was not a cow, or a sheep, or even a horse. It was a llama. The llama farm was in Nidderdale.

Nidderdale is a lovely part of North Yorkshire, but quite different from the llama's natural home in the high Andes. However, the llamas seemed to thrive here. Their role is much the same in North Yorkshire as it would be back in their native South America. The llamas of Nidderdale are *trekking* llamas.

Visitors can fill panniers with picnic blankets, pork pies and Prosecco and enjoy a happy wander with a laden llama, to the heather-clad tops of Nidderdale and around the eerie outcrops of Brimham Rocks. It is rather different from a classic ramble or a traditional pony trek and is a fantastic way to spend an afternoon.

I had nipped home from the surgery for lunch – oh, the joys of living close to work! This was one of the advantages of traditional rural practice and made up in some measure for the endless hours on call and the disrupted weekends. I could walk the dog, put the washing out or stoke up the fire before Anne got home later in the evening. When the boys were small, it was precious extra time with them when most dads would be at work until bedtime. Today though, my lunchtime relaxation was short-lived. My phone was ringing.

'Julian, are you busy?' asked a mildly agitated Sylvia. 'I've just had Suzanne on the phone. She has a llama called Dobbie with a damaged face. She says there's blood everywhere and it sounds nasty. I know you've got afternoon surgery, but it's quite urgent. Can you go?'

Sylvia was efficient, intuitive and a joy to have as a right-hand woman in charge of reception. Her job was often difficult – endlessly busy with a stream of concerned owners, both at the desk and on the phone. She coped so well because of her eternal and youthful enthusiasm, which was infectious. She knew that my absence from afternoon surgery would bring her more problems. I had a number of people coming in for follow-up checks and it would be her job to appease them when I wasn't there, but she also knew an emergency when she heard one.

'Okay, I'll go there now,' I said. 'Can you apologise if anyone has come to see me specially, please?'

I could think of a couple of clients who would already be

waiting patiently. One was Rufus the Shetland Sheepdog, a favourite of mine, who had more problems than I could remember.

As soon as I had finished speaking to Sylvia, I phoned Laura, who was one of the producer-directors for *The Yorkshire Vet*. She wouldn't forgive me if I rushed off to see an injured llama without her.

'Hi Laura, sorry to disturb your lunch, but I've got to go and see a llama. There's been some sort of accident and it has an injured face. It sounds like it's been kicked. Do you want to come?'

'Too right I do,' she enthused. 'Where can I meet you? I'm just eating a sandwich, but I can be at the garden centre in five minutes. Would that work? I'll set off now.'

The plan was hatched – the garden centre was on the way to the farm and equidistant from my house and the office where Laura was eating her sandwich. I had soon picked up my camerawoman and we set off for Nidderdale.

As I drove, Laura quizzed me: 'What are we going to see, Julian?' and 'What's the worst thing that could happen?'; but I really didn't know. I dared not elaborate on the very worst thing that could happen – a kick to the face could have devastating and unpalatable consequences. I guessed there was some sort of gash, maybe as a result of a kick. Llamas are lovely and inquisitive animals, but their kicks are well placed, accurate and fast and they do not suffer fools gladly. I thought there would probably be a cut, which would need stitching. Llamas – and their smaller cousins, alpacas – do not like their faces or heads being touched, so I knew I could be in for a struggle and Laura would be there to catch Dobbie's and my anguish.

But Dobbie's injury was much worse than just a skin wound, as Suzanne, the owner of the farm, explained in a rush as we got out of the car.

'It's his face – I think he's been kicked by one of the others. His jaw's broken I'm sure, it's all floppy. I think you'll have to put him down! He's been such a good llama and I hope you can fix him, Julian, but I don't think you'll be able to. Come and look, he's inside here.'

Suzanne, flushed and upset, led me towards the barn where some of the llamas lived.

Sure enough, there was Dobbie, in a terrible mess. I recognised him because I had castrated him a few months earlier. All llamas have distinct personalities and appearances – colour, coat type, face size and shape, ear fluffiness, expression – and Dobbie, despite his bloodied and lopsided lower jaw, was still unmistakable. Even from the other side of the pen, the severity of the injury was clear. The fractured lower jaw was dangling and bloody. I inwardly cursed myself for not speaking to Suzanne before I left the practice. Had I realised that this might have been the problem, I would have brought some orthopaedic wire with me. If I was going to do anything to help Dobbie, I would have to do so with the equipment I had in my car boot. It was a long journey to their farm and it would be impractical to go back to Thirsk for extra kit.

We ushered Dobbie into the handling pen. It was made especially for restraining llamas, with a multitude of straps to keep the animal stationary. Once restrained, the llama was immediately calmer. I refrained from making an ill-timed joke along the lines of 'Look – now the llama is calmer. I'm-a-poet-and-I-didn't-know-it', since I had come to realise that Laura would be sure to catch it on camera. I have learnt this the hard way, because many of the slightly flippant comments I have made as asides have ended up in the middle of *The Yorkshire Vet*.

There were no jokes to be made today, because everyone was worried – Suzanne about the future of one of her favourite llamas, Dobbie about his painful and floppy jaw and me about what on earth I was going to do to fix it. Vets are very good at adapting to their circumstances. This is part of our training. For example, we don't need to learn the detailed anatomy of every single species of animal. Rather, we learn the anatomy of the dog in detail and about the intestinal system of the ruminant and then we learn the differences between these and everything else. It is called *comparative anatomy*. We are taught to apply first principles to every situation and, in that way, we can work out an appropriate course of action, even if we have not treated that particular condition or type of animal before. So, while I had never repaired a fractured jaw in a llama before (and as far as I can remember, there wasn't even the smallest mention of camelids when I was at vet school), I had repaired the same injury sustained by countless cats in the aftermath of not quite dodging a passing car. Although Dobbie's face was ten times bigger than a feline face, I planned to carry out a very similar procedure. Maybe I could call it *comparative fractured jaw repair*?

I rummaged around in my disorganised car boot and found the strongest nylon I had. This would usually be used to suture the thick skin of cows, after a Caesarean operation, for example. Today though, I was planning to use it to make something like a set of dental braces. My idea was to loop it around the teeth on either side of the fracture line, to pull the broken bones of Dobbie's jaw into position. I could also pass the thick nylon through the rubbery parts of the gum with a needle, to encircle the whole front part of the jaw. In this way, I hoped the jaw would regain its stability, giving at least some sort of temporary relief until I could come back with my proper wire.

I explained my plan to Suzanne, who was almost in tears with gratitude. She had been certain that Dobbie would have to be euthanised. Laura, still with her camera, was equally delighted – the case had all the makings of a fantastic story.

I set about injecting local anaesthetic into all the areas where I would need to put needles. Slowly but surely my loops of nylon, which were mostly placed around the base of the incisor teeth, were beginning to pull the broken pieces of jaw back together. Not all the sutures were successful and I had to take one or two out and try again, but after half an hour or so Dobbie had regained a relatively pain-free smile of which he could be proud. Well, proud-ish. Unperturbed by the ordeal, he was soon back at his hay net, testing out his new face.

He had been a model patient and I bade him and his owner a relieved farewell, promising to return before too long with my wire in case a more robust repair was required. As we drove back over the undulating road from Pateley Bridge back towards Ripon, with the Yorkshire Dales behind us, the late-winter sun clung on, illuminating in the distance the golden scarred crag of Whitestonecliffe above the village of Sutton and highlighting the White Horse of Kilburn, just to the right. For me, both of these sights signified home. I would be late for evening surgery, but that didn't matter. It felt good to have been doing what I loved. Laura was buzzing: 'That was totally amazing!' she kept repeating, as she scrolled back through the footage on her camera screen. 'You've saved his life! It's just brilliant. What an afternoon! Thank you so much!'

As we chatted happily all the way home, watching the glow on Sutton Bank deepen to ochre, then fade completely, I wondered whether, maybe, the future wouldn't be so bad after all.

If repairing a llama's jaw wasn't an unusual enough case to be dealing with, slap-bang in the middle of calving and lambing time, then Fiver the lamb certainly was. Katy, a superb young veterinary surgeon who had recently joined the practice at Thirsk and whose father had a sheep farm towards York, sidled up to me one evening after consults were complete.

'Julian,' she said, in a manner suggesting either that she had made a big mistake and needed to confess, or that she had a favour to ask. I guessed she was looking to swap a weekend on call, but was very surprised by what came next: 'My dad had a lamb born the other day. It's got five legs. Apart from that, the lamb's fit and healthy, but its extra leg is sticking out of the front of its shoulder. It looks ridiculous, but it's not causing any harm. Dad's worried that it will get in the way as the lamb grows older. Do you think we could take it off?'

I'd never seen a live lamb with five legs, let alone done the procedure. I could sympathise with Katy's dad's dilemma. She showed me some pictures of the lamb on her phone. It did look ridiculous and bizarre and the weird, vestigial extra appendage was sure to cause problems. It did, however, look feasible to remove.

'You know what, Katy,' I declared. 'I think we should give it a go. It's no good having a lamb with five legs and if it's fit and well otherwise, I think we should do what we can.' Sensing the next question, I added, 'We'll just charge for the anaesthetic, so it won't cost a fortune. And we can do it together – I bet you've not amputated a leg before? I'll show you what to do and help if you want.' Vets have businesses to run for sure, but we also have a duty of care. A duty of care to the animals for which we are entrusted and to the community – farmers, pet-owners and horse folk – around the area. It would have been unreasonable to make the cost of saving this little lamb's life prohibitively expensive. That is how I've always worked, as does any practice that values the heritage of a veterinary surgery in a rural community.

'Thank you, Julian,' Katy said and skipped off excited at the prospect of saving this little lamb and learning a new procedure.

Fiver arrived the following day. Once again, Laura was on hand, smiling constantly as usual. If this went to plan, she would have yet another bumper story to add to her list and to cheer up the production and edit team of *The Yorkshire Vet* back in Leeds.

The lamb looked pretty healthy, apart from the extra leg protruding from its right shoulder area. It was pointing forward, just as an umpire would to indicate a batsman needed to make his way back to the pavilion. I'd never seen anything like it and, for the second time in not very long, I found myself relying on experience, drawing on previous sheep anaesthetics (not many) and previous limb amputations (plenty). As with Dobbie, there had been no lecture at vet school on 'How to Amputate the Fifth Leg from a Young Lamb', but it was fine – comparative anatomy in action again. This time I had Katy to help, too. It offered a good opportunity to teach her some surgical skills – she could do the op while I lent a hand and gave advice.

Everything was going smoothly. Fiver was asleep, the area was clipped and prepped and Katy had made her first incision. Suddenly the little lamb stopped breathing. The nurse acted quickly, starting to ventilate with oxygen.

'Is it okay if I take over?' I asked Katy, sensing her starting to panic. We got the little lamb breathing again and, as swiftly as I could, I removed the extra limb. Within a few minutes the skin and muscles were re-sutured, and Fiver was lifting her head and looking around, trying to work out what had just happened. The tension in theatre evaporated the moment she let out a tentative 'baaa', and we all felt glad we'd had the courage to tackle the job.

I've called in at the farm a couple of times since Fiver's operation to check on her progress. After her fleece had regrown, it was impossible to tell her apart from the rest of the flock. More recently, as her fame extended across the county – thanks to her appearance on television – I visited her again. The local news ran a feature on her. By that time Fiver was fully grown and not quite so cute, but her story was no less amazing.

I'd seen some remarkable cases this spring and I was loving my job more and more each day. For all its ups and downs, for the moment at least the life of a Yorkshire vet was a good one!

4. Neville the not-so-wild Boar

'Julian, I need your help,' declared Lisa down the telephone. Lisa was a pig farmer I knew well. She kept a herd of woolly pigs, called Mangalitzas. They were covered in thick hair and, from a distance, with their curly cream-coloured woolly coats they could quite easily be mistaken for sheep. Close up, it was a different matter as they could be rather ferocious. My favourite was a sow called Monica. The first time I met Monica, she had just delivered her first litter of piglets. Things had gone smoothly and my job was simply to check that she had finished and to administer an injection of oxytocin, to help expel any afterbirth that might still be attached. A couple of days later though, things were not so good. Monica had lost her appetite. She wouldn't even touch melon or banana, which were her favourite treats. I was called out again to check her over. This time, the sow was less than amenable to examination. She was fiercely protective of her beloved baby balls of squeaking cotton wool and the minute I set foot in the sty, she charged angrily and extremely fast towards me, tusks bared and saliva flying. It was a close call

– I just managed to escape through the gate before a disastrous encounter between her tusks and my leg. In the end, I managed to inject her using a syringe mounted on a long lance and luckily this did the trick, but I was left with a healthy respect for the fearsome Mangalitza.

Today's phone call, unusually, was not about one of the woolly herd. It was about a new piglet, called Neville. He was due to arrive on the farm in the next few weeks. He was not just any pig, as Lisa went on to explain.

'He's just a few weeks old,' she said. 'He was found on a road in the Forest of Dean. He had no mum, so we think he must have wandered off and got lost in the woods. He's at a rescue centre at the moment, but he needs a new home and I think he'll fit in well here with us. The rescue centre was based just outside the Cotswolds – an area almost as beautiful as Yorkshire itself – and was adept at coming to the rescue of wildlife of all shapes, sizes and species. While they were capable of caring for injured owls, under-weight hedgehogs and the occasional badger, a wild boar – even a small one – would be too hard to look after. Neville, the not-so-wild-boar, needed a new home. Chris and Hilary, the managers of the centre, looked for help and Lisa answered their call. The thing is, he is a *wild boar*. He's happy where he is at the moment, but they can't keep him because they don't have pigs and besides, he's already starting to get big. Before long he'll need to be somewhere with other pigs – you know, to keep him company.'

I listened with interest and surprise. I conjured up an image of Neville the baby wild boar, having sauntered away from his pig family, standing by the side of the road waiting for a bus to take him to the rescue centre; or perhaps the shopping centre; or the swimming pool; or even the swings. It was the stuff of children's stories.

The actual story of Neville's arrival at the rescue centre was not too far removed from the imagined story in my mind. He *had* been found, lost, near a bus stop in a wooded area on the edge of a little town. A family had taken the little pig to the local centre, who immediately identified him as a wild boar. The implications of this were significant. Neville, cute as he was, would quite quickly grow into a big pig and this would bring with it significant problems. An adult wild boar would be a very different proposition from the stumpy little character rescued from the roadside. Neville would become difficult to manage. If he were to be rehomed, he would need to go to a farm that could deal with such creatures.

'It's like this, Julian,' Lisa continued. 'A friend knew I had my herd of unusual pigs and put the centre in touch with me. Poor little man needs a home and I'm sure he'd fit in here. What do you think?'

I pondered the situation.

It is not every pig farm that would welcome a wild pig into a healthy herd, as Lisa was planning to. The newcomer might carry disease. He might upset the locals. He might just not fit in. He might be actually wild. But, I knew that Lisa was kind and caring and always happy to help an animal in a pickle. Neville was certainly in a pickle and there was no doubt that Lisa's farm would make a lovely home. I explained the health risks, but knew Lisa's love and caring nature would prevail and that she would be able to take the appropriate measures to minimise these risks. But there was one other big dilemma with Neville's arrival.

'The other problem,' I went on, trying not to sound too negative, 'is that a wild boar, even a baby one, is classed as a *dangerous wild animal*. I know he won't look like a dangerous wild animal right now, but you'll need a special licence from the council to keep him. You'll have to fulfil various criteria for them to grant you a licence and they are pretty strict. I can come and do an inspection and fill in the forms if you like. It takes a few weeks to process the paperwork, but it should be straightforward. Please remember, though, he will turn into a big pig and he might be a handful.'

Lisa was unperturbed by the potential problems or the paperwork.

'Julian, he just needs a new home. We managed to deal with Monica, remember? After her, he can't be that bad, can he?'

And with that, and with the recollections of past encounters in my head, I agreed to start the process that would enable Neville the wild boar to make his home in North Yorkshire.

A few weeks later I rounded the hairpin on the way up Sutton Bank, and headed up across the moors towards the coast. The temperature fell its customary three or four degrees as I reached the top of the bank and the grey light of Thirsk was replaced by a thick fog that hung in great swathes, like the inside of a cloud. I was on my way to visit Lisa's farm. Even though I had looked after her pigs for years and knew the farm well, I was still required to inspect the premises for its suitability for keeping Neville the new *dangerous wild animal*. I was used to doing these inspections for the local council. As well as wild boar, ostriches, American bison and camels are also classed as *dangerous wild animals* and a few farms nearby kept these creatures. It is a sensible move to require licensing, as it is crucial that these species are handled and managed safely and also that the public is kept safe. It would be no good if wild pigs escaped and rampaged through the local villages or through local farms. I couldn't imagine which of the animals on the list would be most alarming, if any of them escaped. A stray camel would certainly get heads turning down the streets of Easingwold, but I think an American bison would be fairly scary!

Sometimes, inspections involve not just the vet, but also an environmental health officer, whose job is to check important documents like insurance, public liability and so on. Today though, the local authority decided that, working from their checklist, I could manage on my own. I jumped out of the car, pulled on my wellies and grabbed a clipboard.

My first job was to draw a map of the farm. It wasn't very good – I am, after all, a vet and not a surveyor: my lines were not straight and it was pretty rubbish if I'm honest, but it would have to do. Next, I moved onto the actual inspections. I checked the electric fencing and gates to make sure the new pig could not escape; I checked the food stores to make sure they were clean and hygienic; I checked movement records and medicine books. Everything was in order, as I knew it would be – Lisa was an excellent farmer – so I moved inside to look at the barn where Neville would be spending the first few months of his new life at this haven for pigs. I turned over the page of my checklist. To my surprise, the next page of questions asked for details of the inside housing. I read and reread the questions:

'Is there sufficient bedding in the housing?' Yes, there was. The yard was deep with straw that would be perfect for a pig.

'Is the space adequate for the **dangerous wild animals**?' Indeed. The fold yard where Neville would be living was spacious. I paced it out for an approximate size and made notes on the form where necessary. Once summer arrived, Neville would be in a field, surrounded by electric fences so he couldn't escape. But even in the winter housing area, there was definitely plenty of space.

'Is there adequate furniture for the animal?' I looked at Lisa as I read out this question. The straw bale that I was sitting on was certainly comfy, but whether it could be described as furniture was a different matter. After some thought, considering the type of furniture that a baby wild boar rescued from the woods would need, I ticked the box. Yes, the furniture *was* adequate.

Next question: '*Are there sufficient play items for the **dangerous wild animal**?*'

I raised my eyebrows at Lisa. This form-filling exercise was beginning to sound silly. I wondered who had designed it, suspecting it had been adapted from the paperwork used for puppies or maybe even children and that, back in the council offices, there had been one 'copy and paste' too many.

'Well, apparently Neville does like to play football,' said Lisa. 'I've got one ordered for when he arrives.'

I ticked the box and signed at the bottom of the page. Lisa's farm had passed my part of the inspection. Now we had to wait for the council to approve the paperwork. I hoped they were happy with my assessment, despite the possible contentious nature of the furniture and playthings.

Then it was just a matter of arranging a time for Neville to arrive. Once again, my imagination ran wild – I had visions of the perky little piglet hitching a lift or getting off the coach in the middle of Thirsk. However, there was one more important consideration.

Lisa's herd was healthy, free from disease and miles away from any other pig farms. A new pig of uncertain provenance, found in a wood, could bring in disease. I advised that he should be tested before he arrived. I couldn't tell how healthy he was from three hundred miles away, but I had discussed what tests were needed with the veterinary surgeon who looked after the rescue centre where Neville was staying. He wasn't so sure that blood-testing a piglet was his department. It was a far cry from tending to poorly hedgehogs and concussed owls.

But, after several reassuring emails and a long conversation, Neville successfully donated a couple of millilitres of blood to be tested – nearly a whole leg-full for a piglet. Sadly, this was not the final hurdle. When the lab received the tiny sample of Neville's blood to check it for diseases, concerns were raised: 'It's not a very good idea to accept a wild pig onto a breeding unit, you know?' commented the laboratory vet, who was an expert in pig husbandry. I did know this. It was the reason I had asked for the blood tests in the first place. The laboratory vet must have assumed Lisa's pig farm was a concrete-clad, intensive unit, with fast-growing, super-lean, super-sensitive, modern pink pigs. But the robust Mangalitzas were a very different type of creature altogether. Yes, they were still prone to problems of disease, but the extensive, mainly outdoor, hard-as-nails, traditional hairy pigs would not be fazed, hassled or intimidated by Neville – either as a small piglet or when he became a large boar. They would give as good as they would get and, assuming freedom from disease, Neville would fit in a treat.

The wait for the blood results and the wild animal licence was tense. Eventually, both came back with positive news. The blood tests for all the diseases a pig can get were all negative. Neville was in the clear. The council also agreed to play ball and the licence was issued. So, soon Neville would be playing with a ball of his own, in a straw-filled fold yard in the middle of the North York Moors.

My daydream of Neville arriving by coach didn't materialise. He came in a trailer, pulled by a car. I made sure I was around when he arrived. Everyone was excited. Lisa was excited to meet the long-awaited piglet. The people from the rescue centre were excited to see his new home and to give their thanks to Lisa, who had saved this little pig's bacon, so to speak. And me – I was excited to see Neville's reaction to his new surroundings. And of course, I wanted to see how good he was at football.

The car and trailer pulled into the farmyard, which was spotlessly clean – Lisa had made a special effort. The pen where Neville was going to make his home – in fact, his living room, given the furniture – looked comfortable, deep in fresh, clean straw. We all held our breath as the trailer door came down, the gates opened and Neville the not-so-wild-boar emerged, snuffling and shuffling all the way down the ramp.

'I've put him next to Laura – the pig over there in that yard,' Lisa called to Chris and Hilary, the devotees who spent their lives helping stricken animals. The fact that they had spent a day delivering an eight-week-old piglet to the depths of North Yorkshire was testament to their dedication and commitment to the job that they clearly loved.

'She doesn't have many friends. She's got a bent nose so the other pigs bully her,' Lisa went on to explain, pointing to Laura, the woolly pig on the other side of the fence.

'I think they'll get on like a house on fire. I'm going to let them sniff each other for a few days first, then I'll let them mix. In the meantime, Neville, here's your new football.'

Lisa was doing her best to reassure Chris and Hilary that Neville would be fine.

'Thank you so much for having him, Lisa,' said Chris, who was obviously sad to see the piglet go, but glad that this would be the perfect place for a boar like Neville. As he grew older, he would need to be in a suitable environment – safe and stimulating. Chris knew he had everything he needed here.

We leant against the gate of the yard, watching the piglet get used to his new surroundings, his roommate, his sofa and his football. It was a happy time. I could have lingered but I had more visits to make – the rest of the day would be filled with more conventional veterinary work!

As I said goodbye to everyone and shook Chris's hand, he added a final few words of advice: 'I know he's *called* a wild boar, but just remember, he's not really so wild at all.'

I was already looking forward to my next visit. Neville and I might even get to have a kick-around!

5. A Bee Sting in the Eye and Christopher Nibbles

During my time working as a veterinary surgeon I've seen many different animals. With the exception of zoo animals, I've probably seen most things. For the last few years, I've also been involved with the making of the Channel 5 programme *The Yorkshire Vet*, which has been a fantastic opportunity to share the work of a mixed practice with anyone who cares to watch. The remit of the show (an entertainment programme, not a documentary, as I am occasionally reminded by the series producer), is both to showcase the beautiful Yorkshire countryside and to embrace, quite literally, all creatures great and small. The variety of animals and people that we encounter in mixed practice provides the warmth and character for each episode and is key to the programme's popularity. Just as James Herriot's tales have, at their heart, not just the animal but also the personality of its owner, our programme focuses on the human stories behind every case. Sometimes, in the hectic day-to-day life of the surgery, as we rush from theatre to consult room, X-ray machine to farmyard and back again, it is possible to focus just on the animal, and the next animal, and then the next again. But, behind every sick cat, rabbit or hamster is an owner who also needs our care and attention. They may be worrying about the outcome of a thermometer reading, blood test or X-ray, or anxiously awaiting a phone call about the success or otherwise of an operation. Being involved in making the programme never fails to remind me of the importance of spending time listening to the human behind the animal. Mending the animal often mends the owner, too.

One case I saw, in the early days of filming *The Yorkshire Vet*, stuck in my mind more than most. It was late April and Fudge the cat was suffering from a sore eye. He'd been in a couple of times over the previous few days, but the eye was still bothering him. Fudge belonged to Tommy, a young lad of, I guessed, ten or twelve. Tommy and his mum, Karenza, came in at the end of evening surgery. I was in a rush – I was supposed to be taking Archie, my youngest son, who was an accomplished swimmer and budding triathlete, to one of his first open-water swim sessions. He was waiting patiently for me to finish evening surgery. It was half an hour until we were due to squeeze into our wetsuits and plunge into a murky and certainly chilly lake. It would be a close call which of us would complete the fifteen-hundred-metre loop first – even at his tender age he was much faster than I was, but I hoped I still had the edge over an endurance course. However, I still had to deal with Fudge's eye and, if it turned out to be complicated, we'd be late for our swim. As I looked at the eye my heart sank. It was hugely swollen and looked very sore. I realised that I would either have to risk getting a speeding ticket on the way to the lake or Archie would be late again. Or both.

'It's my little cat – well, he's Tommy's cat really,' explained

Karenza. 'I've been in twice already but his eye isn't getting any better despite these drops. The poor chap can't even open it now.'

I asked a few questions, keeping it brief – yes, confirmed Karenza, it had come on very suddenly. One minute he'd been fine, the next his eye looked like this.

Then, I set about examining the ginger tom. Sure enough, the tissues around the right eye were swollen and oedematous – so much so that I couldn't even see the surface of the eye. It demanded a closer look. Even though it was obviously very painful, Fudge was remarkably calm, continuing to purr constantly. Ginger toms are notoriously relaxed and unfazed!

'I'll need to anaesthetise him, so I can examine the eye in more detail,' I said. I sensed Karenza and Tommy's anxiety over the lack of improvement so far. 'Is that okay? I'll do it now; I think we need to sort it out as soon as we can.'

Tommy stroked his cat's head before he reluctantly persuaded him back into the basket so I could take him through to theatre. The young lad was obviously very worried about his beloved cat and tears were beginning to well up in his eyes.

'Don't worry. I'll look after him,' I reassured, although I wasn't convinced this offered much comfort to the boy.

Before long, Fudge was asleep and I was trying to work out what to do. Archie climbed onto the neighbouring table in theatre to watch. It was a perfect seat from which to spectate. I was expecting to see a grass seed, hiding behind Fudge's third eyelid. These troublesome things are a real nuisance for cats, dogs and vets through spring and summer. With their pointy ends and barbed sides, the seed heads cling on tenaciously. The barbs prevent them from falling out once they have become embedded in or under delicate tissue and they can even penetrate skin. They often get stuck in ears, causing acute distress and manic head-shaking, or between toes, causing oozing sores. I've even seen them inhaled. As they migrate through the lung tissue, invisible to X-rays, they cause terrible pneumonia, mostly in springer spaniels who tend to dive through fields of wheat or long grass. Months later, an abscess-like swelling appears behind the ribs, and when you cut into it with your scalpel, the pesky grass seed pops out, having wreaked havoc through all the internal organs in its path.

I placed little 'stay' sutures in Fudge's upper, lower and third eyelids to allow me to retract them carefully so I could look at the eye underneath. Even under anaesthetic, with Fudge immobile and unaware of my probing, it was hard to examine in much detail because everything was so swollen. The third eyelid in dogs and cats is an extra level of protection for the eye. It extends outwards across the eye from its inner corner, at the bottom. It protects the eyeball from damage by sticks, prodding twigs or scratches from other animals but, occasionally, a grass seed gets lodged under it and this is very painful. However, as much as I searched, I could find no offending grass seed in Fudge's eye. Archie kept looking at his watch, losing interest in the operation when he realised nothing dramatic was about to happen, but very much interested in how soon I would be finished.

Eventually I caught a glimpse of a tiny brown foreign body, sticking into the outer surface of the swollen third eyelid. I carefully grabbed it with flat-ended forceps and pulled gently. Out came a sting – a sting from a bee! I couldn't imagine a worse place to have been stung. There was no wonder the poor eye was so inflamed and painful.

'Ta da,' I exclaimed, raising the almost invisible speck of brown sting into the air with a flourish, relieved to have finally found and solved the problem. Archie didn't look impressed by the tiny object.

'Can we go now?' was all he could say.

'Not just yet, but soon,' I promised. I still needed to instil a tiny amount of steroid into the inflamed tissue to suppress the reaction to the sting. I sent Archie to the pharmacy to get some, with instructions about what it was called and where the small bottle lived. The swelling would settle down now that the sting had been removed, but the injection, with its anti-inflammatory effect, would bring about a more rapid improvement.

'Is this it?' asked Archie when he returned from his mission, holding out the tiny bottle for me to inspect.

'It is,' I confirmed. 'Thanks. Now, please can you shake it for about thirty seconds and then get a 1ml syringe and a blue needle?'

My youngest son had seen a lot of veterinary procedures and he knew exactly where these things could be found. I couldn't help wondering if we had a budding vet in the making. I was sure he would be very good. I would encourage him if this were the path he chose to follow, but I wouldn't try to persuade him. The veterinary profession has changed dramatically over recent years, making it a much more challenging career choice for young people than it has been in the past. While it can be a wonderful way of life, it is not for everyone. Archie had seen both sides of the profession – the satisfying rewards when a patient is cured and the owner happy, but also the nights and weekends on call, and of course the unpredictability of home-time, which made it difficult to get to evening activities with any kind of reliability. This evening was a case in point.

Fudge was soon back in his kennel, resting comfortably on a fleecy bed. He would be staying in the practice overnight, to let my tiny injection do its work and to let him sleep off his anaesthetic. My final job, before heading to the lake, was to call Karenza with the good news and to reassure Tommy that his cat would be fine. I love passing on the happy news of a successful diagnosis and cure. Everyone was delighted and relieved.

Archie and I made it to the lake with minutes to spare. A late-evening open-water swim with my son was the perfect way to end a busy day.

By morning, Fudge's eye looked immeasurably better and he could go home, with instructions to continue with a different type of eye drops.

When I called him into my consulting room a week later for a check-up, Fudge was a normal cat with a normal eye and Tommy was like a different boy. He had a huge, beaming smile as he carefully placed his cat's basket on the table. He'd assumed all the responsibility for applying the all-important eye drops and couldn't disguise his pride in the outcome.

'Tommy has been amazing, Julian,' his mum said, as proud of him as he was with his achievements. 'He faithfully put the drops in, three times a day, just as you'd said. I think we have a young vet in the making! Thank you for fixing Fudge and thank you for inspiring my son. He's hoping to be a great vet one day.'

Some weeks later, there was another young vet-of-the-future with a patient in need of my attention.

Finlay was sitting patiently with his dad, with a box on his lap. His legs dangled from the chair and his feet didn't touch the ground. A small boy with a dad and a box could only mean one thing. The camera crew knew this too and Laura, who was filming today, had already collared this case for me.

'Julian.' She had smiled persuasively. 'There's a boy called Finlay in the waiting room with his hamster. Can we put him on the list for you to see? I'm not sure what's wrong with his hamster, but we'd like to film him, just in case it turns out to be something interesting.'

I nodded. Laura had an uncanny knack of encouraging complicity. When she used terms like 'just in case', it could mean anything from 'just in case it's a spectacularly interesting case of rare-and-peculiar-hamster-illness' to 'just in case the fluffy-but-rather-angry child's pet bites the vet' or 'just in case the kid turns out to say something really funny or really cute'. Whichever way, I knew it would be me treating the small furry animal inside the box this busy afternoon, rather than any of my colleagues. I didn't mind, though. I love hamsters. And guinea pigs, for that matter. It's not what every vet says. But I think hamsters are cute and funny in equal measure and, although they can be adept at sinking their teeth into a vet's finger, I like them a lot – especially if they don't bite me.

I called them in: 'So, who do we have in this box?' I asked. It seemed the right thing to say, rather than my usual 'So, what seems to be the problem today?' I hoped it would engage the young owner and get him to talk me through the case. A shy child, or one who is more interested in playing on his phone than in the small furry in the box, will ignore my questions, leaving the parent to do the talking, but a keen and engaged child usually takes charge, which is better. That is exactly what happened today.

'This is Christopher Nibbles,' explained Finlay, confidently.

'Hello Christopher Nibbles. I'm pleased to meet you,' I said, peering through the small holes in the lid of the box. I wanted to see what I was dealing with before I ran the gauntlet of handling the fast little creature with sharp teeth.

'What's the problem with Christopher Nibbles?'

'His skin has gone all wrinkly and his hair has fallen out. He looks horrible,' replied Finlay, screwing up his face as if to confirm how ugly his pet had become.

'Oh dear, that doesn't sound very nice,' I concurred. 'We'd better have a look.'

I lifted the lid to get a closer look at the tiny patient, before adding, 'Is Christopher Nibbles very friendly?'

'Oh yes, he's a very friendly hamster,' confirmed Finlay.

I looked to his dad for reassurance.

'Well, usually he is fairly friendly,' said Dad, 'But he's not very happy at the moment. He doesn't like travelling in this box and he's bitten me before. I'd be careful.'

It's not terribly easy to examine a hamster. They are fast and too small to make an extensive examination. Luckily for me and for my examination, Christopher Nibbles' problem was easy to see. He had a severe case of dermatitis, causing sore patches and baldness over most of his body. It looked nasty. I gently cupped him in my hands. This was uneventful – Christopher Nibbles showed no signs of wanting to sink his long teeth into my thumb.

'That doesn't look very nice, does it?' I said, trying to confirm the seriousness of the problem without causing too much alarm to Finlay.

I came up with a plan. I gave Christopher Nibbles an injection to help with any infection and then showed Finlay how to apply some thick, white cream to his hamster that I hoped would help to heal the lesions. However, my demonstration wasn't very successful. I misjudged the hamster's small size, leaving Christopher Nibbles looking as if I'd squirted toothpaste on his head. Though he looked ridiculous, he continued to scurry around on the consulting room table, completely oblivious to the large blob of greasy, white cream behind his ears.

'You just do it like that, but try to smear it around better than I have done,' I explained. 'I'm not very good with cream.'

'Okay, I will,' said Finlay, plonking the little, cream-covered hamster back in the travelling box. 'I hope it makes him better.'

As Finlay marched out, I had a quiet word with his dad. I feared that the prognosis for Christopher Nibbles was grave.

Hamsters are prone to a nasty, although slowly progressing, type of cancer that affects the skin. The cream would ease the soreness for a while and give Finlay some extra time with his pet. It would have been a shock to the little boy if I had put Christopher Nibbles to sleep at this early stage, although I confirmed, out of Finlay's earshot, that this would be the likely outcome.

Christopher Nibbles came to see me twice over the following weeks. He looked slightly better at first (allowing me to compliment Finlay on his excellent cream-applying technique) but then quite a bit worse. I explained as gently as I could to Finlay that he wouldn't be getting better. Then the final consultation came. It was peaceful in the end and Finlay was very brave.

Laura had been filming the hamster's progress throughout, 'just in case'. She went to see Finlay and his dad at home a few weeks later, to ask him questions about his hamster and his life.

I wasn't there and so I didn't see this interview until I perused the 'rough cut' of the episode in which Christopher Nibbles featured. (I watch all the rough cuts, to make sure everything is accurate. The editing process can distort the clinical accuracy sometimes, as a complicated case is cut to size.) Little Finlay was sad, but had come to terms with the death of his first pet. He concentrated hard as he answered Laura's questions and spoke eloquently about his loss, before finally concluding: 'Christopher Nibbles is in heaven now.'

I felt sure hearts across the nation would melt when this episode was on the telly.

6. TB or not TB, That is the Question

The message in the daybook piqued my interest. It was a request for me to telephone Alan, the senior vet of a neighbouring practice. What would it be about, I wondered? A client moving from one practice to another perhaps? Some local gossip among the veterinary community of North Yorkshire? A reference for an applicant for a job? An idea for some sort of collaboration for the future? It might, of course, just be to borrow a bottle of an unusual or hard-to-come-by medicine. Whichever it was, it sounded much more interesting than some of the other calls demanding my attention, so I picked up the phone at the first opportunity. The call to a client about a dog with chronic diarrhoea could wait for half an hour.

Besides, Alan and I got on well and it was always nice to have a chat and a catch-up. It felt like the old days, two or three decades ago when rural vets generally enjoyed harmonious and cooperative relationships with neighbouring practices.

I dialled the number.

'Hi Alan, Julian here. I'm just returning your call from earlier. Everything okay?'

'Yep,' replied Alan succinctly, 'could do with another vet – overworked as ever – but all is good with us. How about you?'

'Good, thanks. Busy but can't complain about that. How can I help?'

'Well it's this blooming TB-testing business.' I could sense a silent groan. 'It's just not financially viable for us now. I'm not planning to revalidate my testing status. I'm just too busy and, you know, at two quid a cow, it doesn't stack up. But, we do have a few clients who have a bit to do – post-movements and so on. I wondered – if you are still doing it – would you like to do some for us?' Alan was taking the 'generously offering me some work' tack rather than the 'would you like to do the unprofitable work for me' approach, although I knew him well enough to know he wasn't shirking a job. He worked his socks off and, if I could help him, it would benefit both our practices.

A post-movement TB test is a specific type of tuberculosis test, performed on some cattle after they've moved from place to place. It is actually the easier type of TB test to perform. It usually involved following up animals which had moved out of a TB-affected area or following cattle from herds which had subsequently succumbed to this chronic and indolent disease. It was not terribly onerous and so it was easy to agree to Alan's plea for assistance. Besides, it would give me scope to explore new parts of North Yorkshire and meet new farmers. I explained that I *would* be revalidating my TB training. Even vets who were experienced at testing cattle for TB needed to go on a training course every few years to confirm that they were still capable of doing the job. The cost of retraining was irksome at best and, for some practices, prohibitive.

'Okay. No problem,' I agreed. 'Just ask them to give me a call and I'll fix up their tests if I can fit them in. It'll have to fit around my other work, though.'

'Thanks, Julian. That's a real help. We have some great farmers and I think you'll enjoy meeting them.'

And that was it. I wasn't sure quite what I had let myself in for. Only time would tell . . .

It wasn't long before the first of Alan's farmers called me. He was a polite and well-spoken chap called Mike. One of his fields was next to a farm that had experienced a positive intradermal test – the dreaded *reactor* – a situation feared by all cattle farmers. Even though Mike's cattle were nowhere near the actual cows on the affected farm, the rules stated that all his cattle needed to be tested before they could be moved out of their winter shed. The testing needed to be done within a specified time frame and Mike was anxious to get his cows out as soon as the warm and dry weather of spring arrived, and the grass started to grow. Cattle are healthier and happier out at grass than anywhere else.

So, I headed off to an unfamiliar part of North Yorkshire – fifteen miles to the south of Thirsk, deeper into the Vale of York. At this time, I was one of just a few vets to have retained the qualifications to carry out this antediluvian test, which was laborious and tedious in equal measure. It was a similar situation to the one that took Alf Wight, or James Herriot in his famous books, to far-flung parts of the county, TB-testing the cows of Wensleydale. The work he did, many decades ago, provided the characters for his iconic stories. As I drove off into uncharted territory, I felt – more than usual – that I was following in Alf's footsteps.

When I arrived at the farm, Mike, his father, and his daughter Rosie were all waiting for me. Rosie was a would-be vet student and keen to get involved, although the enormous cast on her leg from a recent ligament injury made her less helpful than she might otherwise have been. After a round of introductions, I briefly explained why I was there – the nature of TB-testing in the UK had become more and more complicated, but Mike and his family knew all about it. They were very much 'up to speed' with all aspects of farming and the health of their herd. They had won the coveted 'Beef Farmer of the Year' trophy a couple of years previously and had one of the best, healthiest and most progressive herds in the country. As we ploughed through the perfunctory testing job we chatted, covering many topics concerning the farming and veterinary worlds, and the conversation was inspiring. Mike explained his herd's health and management strategies, including an innovative technique for managing his grassland that protected the delicate substructure of the soil, maintaining its composition and minimising the use of man-made fertilisers. Here was a family totally dedicated to progressive farming and happy, healthy cattle.

Once we had finished the first batch, we moved to a second group of animals in some buildings a mile or so away from the main farm. Mike explained how critical he considered it to interact with his cattle, to talk to them and become 'part of the herd'. But this was not hippy-style anthropomorphism. Mike was a pioneering, groundbreaking farmer who loved his animals and realised that forming a relationship with each and every cow on his farm provided a positive experience for everyone, especially the cattle.

'Come and have a look at these heifers, Julian,' he suggested, as the last of the animals to be tested left the crush. 'They're our yearlings and they are already out getting some fresh air. They're in this field, behind the shed – I'll show you what I mean when I say all farmers should talk to their cattle.'

We went through the gate into the grassy field. The clover was popping through and the lush green shoots suggested winter was behind us and spring had definitely arrived.

'Come on girlies, *shoop, shoop*,' Mike called. Sure enough, just like a group of obedient Labradors faithfully following their master, a gang of about twenty heifers came ambling towards us. Within just a few moments, we were surrounded, each animal jostling to be stroked on the neck and patted on the back. It was truly amazing. Heifers are usually wild and unruly creatures, who would charge either away from you or straight at you. I could not think of any farm I'd ever been to before where this experience would have been possible.

I filled in the paperwork and arranged with Mike to return three days later to read off the test. I'd tested forty cattle or so, spent half an hour talking to some heifers in a field and met an inspiring farming family. It wasn't much of a money-spinner, but I was glad I'd taken up Alan's offer to help out. Treating animals is what vets do, but every animal, every herd and every flock has an owner. In many ways, it is the human aspect of veterinary work that is the most fascinating and I love meeting new people who are passionate about what they do. I couldn't help wondering where my next Herriot-style TB test would take me. If it was going to be as interesting as this one had been, then I looked forward to it.

I was trying to put the question marks over the future of Skeldale to the back of my mind and concentrate on work. Discussions were continuing with a depressing tone (as far as I was concerned and as far as the future of independent mixed practice in Thirsk was concerned). More meetings were scheduled and my partners were planning a trip to see the company headquarters in Watford, three hours south on the train. Phone calls were made to other vets, whose names had been provided by the company, who had recently sold their practices and who, apparently, confirmed that 'yes, it had been a great idea'. Well they would, wouldn't they?

I had done some research. I had checked out the history of the company, their level of borrowing, the venture capital investors who had recently ploughed in a tranche of cash to fuel the purchasing spree. What would they think about TB-testing the friendly cattle of some friendly farmers? Not much, at two quid a head, I imagined.

I'd read reviews written by staff who had worked for the company and I'd seen the faceless avatars on the websites of not-long-purchased practices, where there should have been photos of vets, nurses and receptionists. I could see the vacant posts for 'senior vets' and the series of locums that seemed to appear at every practice. It hardly fitted with the story of 'one happy family'. I had never seen any family photo album with blank silhouettes of family members. I was absolutely sure that this was not the way for me, or my (or at least partly my) practice, to progress. But I could do precious little if my colleagues disagreed with my thoughts.

Whatever I am, I am not a hypocrite. I knew I could not and would not be part of any corporate takeover. I could not continue to work in the practice if the acquisition occurred. I would not be complicit in something with which I so wholeheartedly disagreed. I tried not to dwell too much on the process. It would have sent me mad. It nearly did send me mad. Whichever direction the current negotiations took, I now had no clue what my veterinary future would hold. If Skeldale were to be sold, at this point, I had no idea what I would do next with my career or, indeed, my life.

What I definitely didn't know was that, before many months had passed, I would be working with Alan as a proper colleague, rather than just helping him out of the TB-testing hole that he was in, and I would be working with Mike and his family, caring for his cows on a permanent basis. Within a year of that first TB test, I was grappling with a prolapsed uterus, dangling dangerously out of the back end of one of Mike's best cows, soon after she had calved, at half past one in the morning. We had become good friends. Mike had even invited me to be his guest at a dinner of the historic and deeply traditional Boroughbridge and Aldborough Agricultural Society. Again, without knowing it yet, I would soon become embedded in a new farming community and a new chapter would begin.

7. An Injured Swan and an Alpaca Sex Clinic

U nity was a well-spoken, elderly lady and she was clearly very agitated about her swan. She lived in a picturesque, quintessentially Yorkshire village and had a large pond at the bottom of her garden. In this pond, or rather, on this pond, lived a pair of swans. They were not the benign, domesticated, black variety with red beaks and a gentle disposition but the large, wild, white versions with huge wings and a ferocious determination to avoid human interference.

'Oh, Julian, thank you *so* much for calling me back, I *do* hope you can help me.' She sounded anxious. 'You see, the thing is, I have a swan and I'm worried about him. I have seen you on television and I know that you are a *dab hand* at swans, so I wondered if you'd be able to come and help this one out. He has a bad foot, you see.'

Unity's house was some distance from the practice, but she had clearly decided I was the vet for the job. I have treated a few swans but I am not, by any means, a swan expert. However, I am usually enthusiastic and always keen to tackle a challenge. This enthusiasm goes a long way, which is just as well.

I arranged to visit the swan one afternoon later in the week, between afternoon and evening surgeries. I found the lovely stone-built country house without problems. It had a circular, pebbled area at the top of the drive, which meant I could swoop my car round to point back down towards the gate. This was a habit I had developed over the years. It was a tip passed down to me by a vet called Andy with whom I had seen practice in Skipton as a student. He, in turn, had been given the advice by his one-time boss Donald Sinclair, aka Siegfried Farnon of *All Creatures Great and Small* fame, during his time spent working at the practice in Thirsk.

'Always leave your car ready for a quick getaway!' were the words of wisdom. I think the idea was that, in the event of a disaster on the farm, the hapless vet could escape post-haste and avoid the ignominy of reversing over the neatly kept lawn, the flowerbed or even the cat. I have done this only once (the lawn, not the cat) and it was acutely embarrassing, especially as the visit had not gone completely to plan. My tyres left huge, muddy tracks across the otherwise immaculate lawn as I tried to turn around in a hurry.

It is a tip I that continue to pass on to vet students to this day, although mainly for the pragmatic purpose of saving a bit of time. It is surprising how often the farmer or pet (or in this case swan) owner isn't ready for you when you arrive. A bit of car-manoeuvring gives them time to catch the patient, sort out a bucket of warm water or turn off the telly and put their boots on, without the vet hopping from foot to foot getting agitated that they have five more calls to fit in before evening surgery. Or not . . .

'Thank you so much for coming, Julian,' Unity effused, in much the same way that she had in our previous conversation on the phone. She went on to explain the problem in more detail.

'It's my lovely swan, you see. He's gone a bit lame and, well, I think he has something wrong with his foot. It's fine, of course, when he is in the water, but on land he's not good. I hope you can help. The problem is – well, he's not so easy to catch, you see. I've enlisted the help of my neighbour, Brian.'

So, our patient had not been caught and snuggled up in a shed or a stable as I had dared to hope.

'Hello,' called Brian cheerfully, waving to me as he removed his coat. 'I think we'll be able to catch him in this coat.'

'Okay, that sounds possible,' I said, trying to hide my pessimism. I'd been in this position before, and more often than not ended up with the animal escaping, usually after an hour or so of chasing it about.

'So where is the patient?' I asked, hoping it would, at least, have been penned in a confined area.

'He's on the lake,' Brian explained, without a hint of the despair that had started to creep around the edges of my mind. 'Well, on the island in the middle of the lake, actually!'

'Okay,' I said carefully. 'So how will we get him? Can we tempt him with food, or somehow persuade him to the shore?'

'I'll get in this boat,' Brian declared, 'and row out to the island and catch him there, then bring him to land.' He seemed to have an unswerving confidence.

I planted my hands on my hips as I stood on the bank and watched the rescue attempt, with as much incredulity as frustration at the situation. It was surely never going to work, partly because, even if he managed to grab the swan, Brian would never be able to keep it confined in his rowing boat as he rowed back. Needless to say, the sight of a large man rowing in a zigzag fashion towards him was enough to eject the patient from the island and onto the water. He calmly slid into the now dark lake and swam serenely to the shore, where he stood quietly next to his mate.

Brian arrived back, red-faced through exertion, several minutes later. He was much less serene and in fact rather cross, but even more determined to catch the swan. He leapt out of the boat and rushed at the bird, astonishingly managing to chuck his coat over the swan and pin him to the ground. Success – although the capture had taken us way past dusk and now it was dark, so I examined the bird's troublesome foot with the help of a torch. Luckily, even in the gloom the problem was easy to identify. There was a huge abscess between the toes of the handsome bird, as big as a conker, filling the webbed area completely. It looked painful and distended and needed to be lanced. I gathered some equipment from my car – some local anaesthetic (in case I needed to make a large incision), a wide-bored needle, some surgical-spirit-soaked cotton wool and a scalpel. After cleaning the area thoroughly with the cotton wool, I pushed the needle into the abscess and squeezed gently. Nothing appeared. I was disappointed; I had expected a geyser of pus to explode from the needle. This pus was solid – inspissated. I instilled some local anaesthetic and made a bigger hole with the scalpel. Sure enough, with some more squeezing, solid lumps of yellow, putty-like, cheesy matter started to appear through my incision. The relief that the swan must have felt straight away was very gratifying for everyone concerned. The swan rescue had, against all the odds, been a success!

I gave up on the idea of getting back in time for evening surgery and accepted Unity's kind offer of a cup of tea to celebrate. She was an artist, and showed me some of her work in progress, including a magnificent sculpture of a rhinoceros, as well as numerous half-finished oil paintings.

Several weeks later a colleague, Matt, was called out by Unity again, when he was on duty early one Sunday morning. The lump on the swan's foot had returned. Without Brian around to help, Matt had climbed into the boat himself and manfully chased the swan all around the lake, rowing like a champion but failing to make any contact with the bird at all. Luckily, it made a successful recovery on its own, and we didn't hear any more about it until one day, months later, Unity appeared in the waiting room to see me. In one hand she clutched what was clearly a bottle of wine, while under her other arm was a bigger, squarer, flatter object.

'Julian, I am *so* grateful for your help,' she gushed, 'It was *wonderful* what you did for my swan that evening. By way of a thank-you – I know you liked looking at my artwork – I've made you this . . .' and she gave me the large, brown-paper-wrapped parcel.

I opened it there and then. The parcel contained a beautiful oil painting of the swan floating on the lake. I was deeply touched. It took pride of place in my consulting room for many months and now I have it on my wall at home. It was wonderfully kind and one of the best of the many gifts I'd had. But more of those later . . .

Veterinary surgeons in mixed practice spend most of their time with conventional domesticated animals – cows, sheep, horses, dogs and cats, along with the odd rabbit, guinea pig or hamster – but, somehow, I seem to have the knack of getting roped in to treating an array of unusual animals. Capturing and treating a swan on a lake and being rewarded for this not just with the swan getting better, but with an oil painting, is just one of the mounting number of less-than-run-of-the-mill veterinary encounters I seem to attract.

A few weeks after treating Unity's swan, another unusual veterinary task came my way. I was invited to attend a camelid sex clinic. I work with alpacas and llamas a lot. Both are gentle creatures, utterly endearing and a great pleasure to treat. They have characters and mannerisms quite unlike any other animal, and their owners are usually highly enthusiastic about them, which always makes the work even more enjoyable. In fact, I've been to see some just this morning and being surrounded by a bunch of inquisitive alpacas, peering at me with massive eyes, long eyelashes and each with a different hairstyle and expression in the middle of a snowy field has been a wonderful experience.

One of those enthusiastic owners is Jackie. I have got to know Jackie well over the years and, in truth, have learnt a lot from her. We have developed a symbiotic working relationship – she brings the deep knowledge of alpacas, and I bring the veterinary expertise. On Jackie's farm I've mended young, greedy alpacas who have gorged themselves in the food store, holding them upside down to massage out the rapidly swelling food; I've given plasma transfusions to sick cria (the name for the juveniles), who were short of their mother's natural immunity; I have put down sick patients suffering from incurable diseases; and I have brought new life into the world, untangling tangled legs to deliver brand new alpacas in all their gangly weirdness. I have even performed a fertility test on a stud male, with the unlikely name of Lothario. Sadly, Lothario did not live up to his name and, after our fertility assessment, was retired as a breeding animal and rehomed as a pet.

While I was familiar with many aspects of camelid health, management and welfare, my knowledge about the breeding process was lacking even though Jackie had explained it to me on occasion. So I felt it would be a useful exercise to witness the mating process at first hand. The Royal College of Veterinary

Surgeons insists, rightly, on CPD (Continuing Professional Development). We have to undertake many hours of training, updating or revising skills and techniques, attending seminars and lectures, giving presentations and sharing knowledge. It can be onerous, expensive and time-consuming, often taking vets away from their practice for days at a time. A sunny afternoon with Jackie, learning about alpaca breeding, would be an excellent source of CPD and I was keen to learn from an expert.

I was not completely new to this kind of thing. Any males that were sold as breeding stock from Jackie's farm required a health check. One of the jobs was to assess and measure the penis and measure the testicles of any budding stud male. I was becoming an expert at checking alpaca testicles.

On another occasion, I was called to examine a young female prior to breeding. The young alpaca in question had a persistent hymen, a thin membrane in the vagina that made mating difficult. Under the comfort of an epidural injection it is possible carefully to break this membrane, which is what I decided to do. I had taken the camera crew with me and, as ever, Laura was fastidiously pointing her camera at me and asking questions and I was trying to give a commentary on the process, explaining everything I was doing and why. In an attempt to emphasise the point that this had been a simple and pain-free procedure, I made a comment along the lines of 'I hope the male alpaca will be just as gentle as this when he does his thing.' Just at the very moment those words left my lips, a fly landed on the corner of my right eye. I didn't have a hand free, busy as I still was with the alpaca, so to remove the offending fly all I could do was a rather exaggerated wink. It worked a treat and the fly disappeared. Meanwhile, Laura and Jackie fell about laughing. My wink was timed (or mistimed, depending on your point of view) to perfection and it looked as if I had made some kind of Benny Hill-type innuendo. The clip became part of an episode of *The Yorkshire Vet* but, miraculously, the editing process completely removed the fly!

Anyway, back to the alpaca sex clinic and my CPD. In reality, it was a pregnancy-testing clinic. Unlike many other species, female alpacas will always mate with a male, unless they are pregnant (a pregnant alpaca approached by a male will spin around, spit at him and refuse to sit down). Mating for alpacas is done on the ground. It is very civilised. Today was an exercise in working out which females were pregnant. Ebony, Freya, Florence and Amelia came in, one by one, variously avoiding the enthusiastic advances of the male, whose name was Cosmo. The test is called a 'spit off' and from it Jackie can conclude, with accuracy and speed, which of her girls is pregnant. Since Jackie's females are kept away from the males most of the time, only being mated at specific times – so-called 'hand mating' – she also knows the day of mating and can always work out accurately when they will give birth. It is a very good system and infinitely better than the alternative management system, where males and females run together all the time.

So far, I hadn't seen an actual mating – the girls had all been pregnant. The next alpaca, Camilla, now came into the pen, head held high, looking around with a definite glint in her eyes. Cosmo looked equally excited. Crouching down in the corner of the pen to get a better view, as well as to try to be inconspicuous, much as David Attenborough would do while presenting a natural history programme, I did feel something of a voyeur. Camilla immediately sat down on the straw and Cosmo started making all sorts of excited noises, while maintaining a degree of decorum. He was experienced and had done this before. What happened next was quite remarkable. Cosmo had a sophisticated technique and was evidently an expert on this matter. With his front feet, he massaged Camilla's neck as she looked around, clearly enjoying the experience. Moments later, Cosmo leant forward, while still politely sitting on top of and behind his girlfriend, and whispered words of encouragement into Camilla's ear, first one ear and then the other.

I've watched cows and bulls mating, sheep, pigs and also a stallion at stud. There is lots of thrusting and there is nothing romantic or gentle about the process. But, Cosmo and Camilla could have made a video and sold it as *The Joy of Alpaca Sex*. It was all very tantric. After quite a while – at least quarter of an hour – it was over. Camilla and Cosmo had a kiss and another cuddle and then she was off. It had been an amazing thing to witness. Their gentle and compassionate lovemaking was a great example. Even if it didn't count as official CPD, I'd learnt a lot today. If Cosmo's efficiency was commensurate with his sensitivity, I had no doubt that Camilla would be spitting like a good 'un when she had her next appointment with a male.

8. Plaque Off

This is the fifth book I have written. Writing books has been an amazing experience and an opportunity I never expected to have. I have loved the chance to share some of my veterinary stories and some of the interesting parts of my life with anyone who cares to read them.

As a veterinary surgeon, my work is focused on achieving a result – a diagnosis, a treatment plan, a successful operation. When I go off to calve a cow, for example, the purpose of my job is very clear. I need to get the calf out. A live calf and healthy mum is my goal. Over the last few years though, writing, along with my involvement in creating a television series, has opened up to me a whole new way of thinking, one that I didn't realise was there. It has showed me that there is great merit in doing things that do not have a clear and defined purpose or outcome. Writing a book, or making a Christmas Special episode, ultimately achieves nothing if looked at through the eyes of Julian Norton, Veterinary Surgeon. No lives are saved, no infection cured, no cancer excised. Once upon a time I would have considered the process a waste of time, a trivial irrelevance without any real point or tangible purpose. Now, I realise that there is GREAT merit in making books and programmes that people will enjoy.

Not everyone will enjoy them, of course. Many people probably think a book about the life of a veterinary surgeon in Yorkshire is incredibly tedious. But if just a few people take pleasure from reading my books, or enjoy sitting down to watch *The Yorkshire Vet* on a Tuesday night, then that is a good thing. Bringing pleasure to people is extremely worthwhile, whether it is by means of a book, a poem, a painting, a film or a piece of music. I hadn't quite realised that before 2016 but, in many ways, this realisation has changed my life; or at least awoken a creative instinct of which I was previously unaware.

I have, on the whole, tried to make my books positive and uplifting, while not shying away from some of the low points in my life – notably the tragic death of my close friend Dave, on the Matterhorn in 1993, and the horrendous handling of the foot-and-mouth disease crisis in 2001. This chapter, I'm afraid, is not so positive. If you do not wish to read about my last day at Skeldale, a place I loved, then it might be better to skip to the next one. If you trust me to bear accurate witness, within the constraints of the confidentiality by which I have to abide, then read on. But grab yourself a whisky before you do so.

My final day was tense and sad. Our staff all tried to carry on as normal: the usual greetings at the start of the day; the usual perusal of the daybook to see what was happening; the visits, the ops and, today of all days, meetings to attend. Normal veterinary comings and goings were punctuated by various imperatives for the three partners. There were urgent courier arrangements to make for documents that needed to be signed at the last minute, there were

covert phone calls and urgent appointments to attend, with solicitors and other important people with important jobs to do.

The first meeting was early in the morning, with Brian the
practice accountant, to sort out final details of the accounts.
'Morning Brian,' I said, trying to be cheerful. He followed me
quickly up the stairs to the office, shaking his head with a
grim smile, before putting his fist to his forehead in an expression of the frustration and stress he had been bearing for the
last few months. He had worked tirelessly on our behalf
throughout, and the pressure and fatigue had clearly taken its
toll. Brian and his firm had been the practice accountants for
as long as anyone could remember, but this would be probably
the last work he would do for Skeldale Veterinary Centre. The
new owners would use their own firm, acting on behalf of all
two hundred and fifty-odd branches. It would be more stream-
lined and efficient, apparently. It would also mean another
local business would be put under strain as it lost another
client, another victim of the consolidation of the apparently
fragmented veterinary industry.

It was a tedious meeting but a necessary one and it had to be
completed before lunchtime, so that the final figures could be
agreed upon. Under the circumstances, arguing the toss over a
few hundred pounds of overdue debt, incurred by a farmer whose
cow had suffered a prolapsed uterus in the middle of the night,
seemed futile and irrelevant. I still remember that call clearly,
even though it was about ten years ago. I'd got out of bed, in
the middle of the night in the middle of winter, and saved the
life of the cow, its uterus hanging out of its back end and peril-
ously close to death. But we had never been paid!

Kate, one of the nurses, brought me back to veterinary reality.
'What pre-med shall I use for this little dog? She has a loud
heart murmur.'

I must have looked confused.

'It's for Tess, this collie with the terrible teeth. You booked her in and her owner is hoping you can do the op,' Kate reminded me.

Of course. I knew Tess well. I needed to take X-rays of her chest to check her heart, and then possibly remove the plaque and tartar from her elderly teeth. It would probably be the last procedure I would do at Skeldale and it seemed fitting. I'd known the collie for many years and was good friends with her owners, who owned a beef and sheep farm. I'd looked after their animals, mainly the livestock, for over twenty years and had lost count of the calvings and pneumonia cases I had treated, not to mention the lambings, also too numerous to recount. It was appropriate to be operating on their dog today, of all days.

'I'll come and have a look, Kate. We'd better crack on.'

It was a good excuse to leave the meeting. Brian was capable and committed and knew what he was doing. He didn't need any more help from me. I made him a strong coffee before leaving him to pull at his hair one final time.

I was glad to be back in theatre. The procedure was simple – X-rays and dental. Nothing too taxing, but it was nice to be concentrating on being a vet and to be working with Kate. She was truly one of the best nurses I had ever worked with. Committed and caring, passionate about her job and great fun to work with. We had shed tears over the last few weeks, after the news had been announced about the change of ownership of the practice. We were sad that we were no longer going to be working together, and that everything that was good about the practice was quickly slipping away. But today we just cracked on, enjoying each other's capable company and not talking about tomorrow. We were both best in the moment.

The X-rays showed what we expected – an enlarged heart.

Tess would need to start heart medication. Her teeth were dirty but easy to fix – a scale and polish and so on would be good. I set about removing the plaque with the ultrasonic dental scaler. Before too long they looked lovely. I stood back and admired the result. Tess's teeth were sorted, but she'd need a follow-up check on her heart condition. What should I say to her owners? We'd all been sworn to secrecy about the change of ownership, but I had to say something to friends whom I would not see again. At least, not professionally. I would still see people in town – the town that I had made my home over twenty years ago, where we lived, where my kids were born and had grown from babies to teenagers. What would I say to old clients and friends then?

Kate would have to give Tess's discharge instructions, because once I had finished afternoon surgery I had a meeting with my solicitors in Leeds to go through final details and sign the documents. In a way, I was glad I could do this alone, rather than suffer the ignominy of strained handshakes. A handshake would somehow signal that there were no hard feelings, when in fact I had many.

I treated my final patients: Rufus the Sheltie with his multitude of problems, Pam and her Whippets, Judy with her rescue spaniels, and then headed to Leeds. I knew it would be busy with lots of traffic and I was anxious about where to park. I wanted to minimise any extra stress. Luckily for me, one of the production team from *The Yorkshire Vet* had a camera disc full of 'rushes' that were needed urgently by the editing team at the office in Leeds. 'Rushes' are the raw, uncut bits of filming taken directly from a camera – just another bit of the television terminology with which I had become familiar.

It was fortuitous for me on this afternoon that the need for the 'rushes' to go to Leeds meant that I could get a lift to the solicitors' office, so I didn't have to find a parking space in the city centre. I could come back by train, which was easy from Leeds. I hoped I'd make it back to catch the end of evening surgery. I was hoping to see Sid, and his owner Christine. I'd been treating this complicated cat for his whole life, trying to keep him alive in the face of a string of ailments as he got older. I will tell you Sid's story in a later chapter but for now, suffice to say, he had been an interesting challenge and both he and Christine had become great friends over my time at Thirsk. It would be fitting to see him at the end, so I had asked them to come back that evening, after six as usual, for one final check-up. I wanted Sid to be the last patient I treated at Thirsk. I trusted they'd be brief.

The solicitors were efficient and thorough, but not brief. In some ways, this was a good thing. In another way, it wasn't. I kept looking at my watch, worried I would miss my appointment with Sid. I knew he just needed a simple injection – any other vet could do it – but that wasn't the point. Once it got to half past five, I knew I wouldn't make it back in time for my appointment with my favourite cat. I called Christine's number, but there was no answer. She must have been in the car, probably driving home from work. As I put the phone down, two more solicitors appeared, keen to talk me through important elements of the paperwork. I said 'yes' to every question they asked me, signed the forms and looked at my watch again. It was after six and there was still more to get through. I liked their thoroughness, but I quickly realised I would be there for quite a lot longer. It would then be a ten-minute walk to the station and probably half an hour's wait for a train, and I still needed to collect my car from the practice, where it was sitting for the last time in the car park. I'm not sentimental about cars, but if I had been, I would have been sad for my trusty Mitsubishi right then, patiently waiting for me as it always did, after dark when the rest of the industrial estate had long gone home.

Eventually the solicitors finished their important business. We shook hands and I made my way to the railway station. It was bitterly cold, as stations always are, with a biting wind from the north and a hint of snow in the air. I pulled up the collar on my coat as I scoured the lit-up displays to find my train home. But my mind was battered and I couldn't work out which one would get me back to Thirsk, so I gave up and called Anne, who was so much better than me at finding trains.

'It's all done,' I said, resigned but sort of relieved at the same time.

This was the end of the happiest time of my life, but it did mark the start of a new chapter. A chapter that had yet to be written. Anne told me which train I needed, when it would arrive and on which platform I needed to wait. It was a relief and one less thing to think about. She also promised to pick me up from Thirsk station, which was, bizarrely, the place where this whole sorry process had started for me. 'Don't worry, Julian. It will be fine,' were the words still ringing in my ears. I hoped I could trust them, because so far it didn't feel fine at all.

I got on the train and sent a text message to Anne. *'Can you bring a screwdriver? Actually, two screwdrivers – normal and cross-headed please'.*

Her reply went like this: *'???'*

'You okay?' Anne asked when I got to Thirsk. I nodded. 'Yep, sort of. Can you drop me off at the practice? I need to collect my car.'

I wanted to get it this evening rather than in the morning, by which time it wouldn't be in what I could think of as 'my' car park.

'I've got your screwdrivers. Why do you need screwdrivers?'

'I have to get my nameplate off the wall outside the front door,' I replied. 'Now seems like the best time to do it.'

So, at ten thirty at night, with snow settling thickly on the car park and spindrift stinging my eyes, in the darkness of the last day of November 2017, I unscrewed my nameplate. It left a ridiculous gap below the others, which only served to accentuate the obvious. I returned the screws to the redundant holes. It looked a little tidier.

'That's the second plaque I've removed today,' I thought, remembering Tess's treatment earlier on, trying to salvage some humour from a sad situation. Had Tess got home okay and had Kate fixed a follow-up check for her heart condition? If I'd had any emotion left in me, I'd probably have shed a tear at this point. I rubbed the remaining nameplates with my sleeve and wiped snowflakes from the plate in my hand:

JULIAN NORTON
MA VetMB GP cert SAP MRCVS

I hoped the snow would keep falling for a while, to obliterate my footprints from the car park.

Then I drove home for the last time. Now there were tears.

9. End of One Chapter, Beginning of the Next

The last day at Skeldale had been strange and sad, but it had not been as emotional as I had expected. I think, in retrospect, this was because all my emotions had been drained from me over the preceding six months. The practicalities of the day meant that sentimentality, for the most part, had to be put to the back of my mind.

I found myself in the middle of Thirsk Market Square later the following morning. I don't remember why. I think I had things to do. I didn't usually have free time on a Friday morning – I was usually at work – so I must have been doing something useful with my free time. Shopping, maybe.

By chance, I bumped into Steve and Jeanie Green. They appeared from a little ginnel beside the old-fashioned sweet shop behind the old post office, on their way to the Market Square. I thought how strange it was that it was Steve and Jeanie who I had been to see immediately after I had my first encounter with the two men claiming to be from the dark side, eight months before.

'Jeanie, Steve, I have to tell you something,' I blurted out, not really knowing what I was going to say or how to say it. I hadn't wanted – or been allowed – to tell anyone about the changes before, but now I was free from the shackles of the 'less is more' instructions I had been given.

I told them the news. They were surprised and quite sad, but wished me the best and gave me a hug and a handshake. Then they went shuffling off to finish their shopping, apparently unperturbed by the big changes to the veterinary world of Thirsk.

My next job that day was a journey down the road to the pretty market town of Boroughbridge. Alan had been stifling the news of my arrival for a few months, but this was the morning he was going to tell his staff that he had finally found an experienced, enthusiastic mixed-practice vet to join the team, hopefully for the foreseeable future. Anne, who had worked at the practice years before, when she first came up to Yorkshire, had been working back there again for a few months, filling a gap in the small-animal rota. She had been finding it hard to keep up the subterfuge imposed by the terms of sale. 'They'll think I've been lying to them,' she said anxiously. 'All this time they've been wondering what Alan was going to do about getting a new vet, and I've had to pretend I don't know the plan.'

I wanted to say hello to everyone at the first practical opportunity. It was late morning when I arrived, and I paused outside the Georgian house in the centre of this ancient town, catching a glimpse through the consulting room window. It oozed history and heritage and, although the building was limited in its extent – it had just one proper consulting room, complete with a large, wooden desk that looked as if had been there for many decades, and no car parking space for clients – I sensed some fine veterinary medicine had been practised here over the years. There must have been lots of stories the building could tell. I couldn't help but wonder whether this historic practice would hold the key to my future; would it suit me perfectly and would I fit in? Would its old-fashioned ways be too restrictive for me? To quote the fluffy words from animal rehoming centres, would it be my 'forever home'? Time would tell. I took a deep breath and walked in.

'Hello, I'm Julian, the new vet,' I said with a grin. They knew who I was, because they knew Anne. Also, they had seen me on TV. I went past the reception area and into the heart of the practice. It looked very old-fashioned, like something right out of the Herriot books themselves. Aged, wooden shelves with chipped and worn varnish, covered in bottles of calcium for recumbent cows and ointments for lame horses, filled the middle part of the building, emphasising the central importance of farming and equine work for the practice. There was a box bursting with trochars for relieving bloated calves, stomach tubes for treating horses with colic, ancient punches for putting rings in the noses of stock bulls and cannulae for inserting into the udders of mastitic cows. Other miscellany was piled up on shelves, haphazard and ready for a busy vet to grab on their way out on calls.

I wouldn't be needing the stomach tubes, nor the mineral bottles, just yet – my veterinary skills were not needed today. I just needed to collect some keys and find out when I was expected the following week. I was an experienced vet and I didn't need my hand to be held, as many vets do who start a new job in mixed practice. But my veterinary competence wasn't the main issue causing concern to the staff. The nurses, receptionists and vets had quickly worked out that their new vet was likely to come with a camera crew in tow. They were naturally anxious about the implications of this and what it might mean for them, for the practice and even for this quiet little town. I tried to allay their fears: 'If there's a camera around, all you have to do is be normal,' I reassured them. 'There's no need to worry. Everything will be fine.' My own words echoed inside my head – I had heard them somewhere before.

I had the weekend off, and also the next two days. I had promised to do a lunchtime talk for a Yorkshire-based cancer charity in Malton. It made sense to do this in the small hiatus between jobs. I also had appointments at two local primary schools, who always like a visit from a vet. The first was at the school where my kids had been when they were younger and the other was at the school of a brave little girl called Freya, who had been a fan of *The Yorkshire Vet*. Freya had been diagnosed with leukaemia and had been through several rounds of chemotherapy. Her mum had contacted me to see if I could cheer her up and give her a boost by visiting her in hospital, which I did on a couple of occasions. This was the second or third time I'd been to her school, encouraging kids to work hard and follow their dreams. I'd also been to Freya's funeral. I wanted to do everything I could to help her family and the close-knit community of which they were all part. It wasn't easy, for many reasons, but at least I left the kids chatting away excitedly as they went off to their lunch.

'I want to be a vet when I'm bigger,' I heard from more than one child.

Anne had implored me to have some time off – some time to relax, to take a deep breath and to recharge my batteries. She was completely right. It was exactly what I needed and what I should have done. She also knew me well enough to know this was unlikely to happen. I was anxious to get back into vet action and kick-start this new chapter in my veterinary career. So just four days off it was and then I was back!

I hadn't started a new job for nearly two decades. Although I knew all about making a diagnosis, operating on an abdomen and calving a cow, I couldn't work out the computer system in the new practice, which put me immediately on the back foot. I couldn't even find the syringes. In many ways, I felt like a novice again and it was odd and discombobulating. All the solid things of my career, the things that had become second nature – like using the computer to make my clinical records – had become unstable and unfamiliar.

My very first patient was a memorable one. It was a puppy called Sandy. Not just any old Sandy though. This was 'Sandy 5', the fifth Sandy to be part of this lovely family. He was an eight-week old Border Terrier puppy, only just collected from his previous home in Wales. It was a simple first case and didn't need any real veterinary intervention. He mainly needed lots of cuddles. He was supremely healthy. Again, my main challenge was to find what I needed in the unfamiliar consulting room.

In my head, I had anticipated that it would take a few weeks to get used to the seismic change in my career, leaving Thirsk and restarting, rebooting ten miles down the road. I am a positive person, looking forward with optimism rather than looking backward with regret or sideways for an excuse. That's what I told myself. In reality, as I was to discover, it would take a lot more than a few weeks, or even a few months. It wasn't just the syringes I had to find. I had to find my way around all the farms, I had to make some new friends and I had to make this new practice my home.

I always used to tell young vets a year or so into a job as an assistant that the first year is the hardest. After that, when clients become familiar and when they've become friends, it suddenly becomes much easier and not so much like work. It was an attempt to keep the young vets I'd employed cheerful and engaged as they started to master much of the routine work in mixed practice. Now I was back in that position myself and it was harder than I'd imagined, harder than I remembered.

Despite constantly getting lost, driving round and around the small lanes in a part of Yorkshire I did not know too well, I was more comfortable, especially in my first few weeks, out on the farm. I felt it was crucial to get to know as many farmers as I could, familiarise myself with the ways of their farms, the brothers and uncles who helped out, the type of farming enterprise and so on. In reality, from a clinical point of view it didn't really matter if this farm was in Bishop Monkton, Whixley, or my previous stomping ground of Sutton-under-Whitestonecliffe or Boltby – the problems were the same and I knew exactly what to do about each one.

My very first farm visit was to see a beef farmer called Alan. He had a wonderful herd of cattle – Simmental and Charollais. Alan always had his cows tested to see if they were pregnant at the end of autumn or the beginning of winter. The type of weather was a better predictor of which season it was than the actual date in December in Yorkshire. It could be cold and snowy or damp, wet and mild. Either way, it was an inclement way to spend an afternoon in early December, but my new boss, Alan, invited me along to this annual job. He wanted to introduce me to one of his best farmers, also called Alan – which caused some confusion, especially to me. Helping my new boss with a long and involved pregnancy-testing job was a good idea in all ways. I got to meet the farmer, I had the chance to work out how to use the ultrasound scanner, an essential piece of equipment to give an accurate diagnosis of pregnancy, and Alan had someone to share his work. As it happened, it was easy to use and, for the second half of the afternoon, Alan (vet) leant against the fence, watching me scan each cow, and helped Alan (farmer) round up those still to be tested. It was essential for Alan (farmer) to know which of his beloved cows were pregnant, so he could organise his herd for winter, so today was a big day. Cows were corralled in a pen and ushered down a long and outdoor channel, called a 'race' so the cows could be placed in a cattle crush at the end. This way, Alan or I could insert the scanner into the proper place and diagnose if each cow was pregnant or not.

As the afternoon slipped into darkness, Alan (vet) needed to head back to start evening surgery, so I finished off the job on my own. The afternoon went on and on, and darkness fell on us all with another batch to test. I'd only been out of veterinary action for two days, but I'd forgotten how hard it was! Alan (farmer) got even more animated at that point, fully explaining all the ins and outs of his herd and all its nuances as well as his husbandry, furnishing me with as much information about his cows as he could.

Just as we had nearly finished, one of the last heifers to be tested jumped at the wrong moment and cut her foot on a gate-post. Blood was pouring everywhere and there was a superficial gash near the heel bulb at the back of the foot. It was quite deep but didn't require sutures. A sturdy bandage would suffice. So, under the light of head-torches, the last job of a long afternoon was to bandage the cut foot. It had been a busy day, with lots of cows and an emergency, but as I waved goodbye to Alan, I felt safe in the knowledge that I'd done a decent job – in both 'PDing' his cows and bandaging the foot – and I was sure that making my first farming acquaintance had been successful.

By the middle part of December, lambing season was already under way. Much of the area covered by the practice is in the Vale of York, similar to my old practice in Thirsk, so lowland flocks were plentiful and the early lambing potential of sheep breeds like Suffolks was exploited. These chubby sheep were designed to lamb much earlier than the tougher, more rugged breeds acclimatised to the rough fells, where sheep have their lambs in the springtime.

Even before Christmas, Alan had offered me directions to some of the farmers who I was likely to need to visit while on call. Mr Kepwick was one of them. The main reason I needed directions in advance was that Mr Kepwick was often difficult to understand. When calling out a vet for a lambing, he would gabble his problem so quickly that it was often impossible to ascertain what was going on. Instructions on how to get to his farm were even harder to understand. Needless to say, on one of my first nights on call, I had to make a visit to lamb a sheep at his farm.

'Mr Kepwick here I've got a yow on lambing can you come straight away straight away,' he blurted down the phone, without pausing for punctuation or breath.

'Yes, of course. I'll be about ten minutes. Just remind me again where you are exactly,' I replied. I knew approximately where his farm was, but in the pitch black of mid-December, farms in the dark were not so easy to spot.

'Sheep Hills Sheep Hills that's my farm it's on the left,' he spluttered. Thankfully I knew the village where he lived, but I tried for a postcode (to add security to the directions), which was delivered at breakneck pace. Then the phone went dead.

I set off, armed with his phone number (although I knew he'd be with his sheep rather than waiting by his landline from now until I arrived at his farm) and the postcode. But, I had not had to rely on postcodes and satnavs ever before to find a farm. Getting to know the farms and lanes when I last started a new job required OS maps. Satellite navigation systems had not been invented. I remember, a while ago, seeing a large, handwritten sign, daubed in bright red, streaky paint, at the end of a farm track in Dalton, a small village near Thirsk (and, coincidentally close to tonight's visit) proclaiming NOSATNAV. It always amused me because there was no punctuation and its message was not completely clear. Was it a plea to ban the sophisticated system altogether? One day, when I went down the grassy lane to vaccinate a pony at the farm, I enquired about the reason for the sign.

'It's all these bloody lorries,' explained the farmer, bristling with annoyance, 'trying to get to the industrial estate over there. They come down here and get stuck. I'm sick of having to pull them out with my tractor!' Luckily, technology had moved on a bit since then and I hoped the system in my Mitsubishi would get me to exactly the right place.

But I was not so lucky. Several laps of the village later, I was no nearer to lambing the sheep, mainly because I was no nearer to the sheep. To cut short a very long and rather tedious story of getting lost on the way to a lambing, I eventually found a lane on the left, with a rickety sign on the gate saying SHEEPHILLS. I clambered out to open the gate, pondering whether to close it again or leave it open in readiness for my departure. Discretion being the better part of valour, I drove through, got out and closed it. I didn't want any escapees running out onto the road on my first visit to the farm.

The night was clear, the moon was full and frost was glittering in the moonlight. The long, straight farm track could hardly have been more picturesque. In other circumstances, I would have had a camera crew with me, eagerly grabbing beautiful shots of my arrival and cutaways of the moon. It would have made the best opening to an episode of *The Yorkshire Vet* ever! But I didn't have a camera crew, it was after midnight, a ewe was in distress and a farmer was worried, probably in part because his vet was late. I soon arrived at the top of the lane and could see the stooped, old sheep farmer in the distance, at the edge of an open-sided Dutch barn. The smell of sheep wafted towards me as I got out of the car – the cold air and the mixed aroma of lanolin, fresh hay and newborn lambs woke me up more than a strong coffee would. Mr Kepwick shuffled towards me and I thrust out my hand to make his acquaintance.

'Sorry I'm late. I had a bit of trouble finding your farm,' I explained.

'Not to worry. You're here now, that's the main thing. She's in here. It's a big lamb and, well . . .' the elderly farmer paused as if to apologise, 'I'm not as dexterous as I used to be, you see?' Wistfully he held up a knobbly hand to demonstrate his age-related failings.

'Don't worry about that,' I said. 'I'll get everything sorted. Have you got some water?'

Mr Kepwick was a farmer from the era where warm water, soap and a towel would always be on hand, so I knew it was a redundant question.

'I have, it's over there. I'll get it while you have a look at the sheep. She's in this pen. She's a quiet old girl so she'll just stand for you.'

I found the sheep and waited for the water and antiseptic to clean my hand and arm before I made my first tentative internal investigation. This is the exciting part for me. Obviously, the best bit of a lambing is delivering the lamb, but the excitement is in the first few moments, when I have to use my brain and my experience to picture the situation inside. I have to work out the size of the lamb, the anatomy of the inside of the mother's pelvis, find the head, the legs, work out which is which and sometimes which legs go with which head. Even on a cold, frosty night when I should be asleep, it's a fun challenge. On this occasion, there were no jumbled-up legs, just a large head to manipulate into alignment. For a vet with small hands and years of experience, this wasn't the toughest job in the world, but it was as satisfying as any when the chunky Suffolk lamb landed on the straw and flapped his ears, signifying he was very much alive. There was a second too and, even before I'd finished washing my hands, the sound of bleating young lambs signalled a successful night's work.

As I looked at the large pen of expectant mothers and the small pens of new lambs, all lit up by the full moon, I realised that Mr Kepwick had only just started lambing. I sensed that this would not be my last trip to Sheephills. But that could only be a good thing. It was a special place and one I felt sure would become a place full of healthy lambs and happy memories.

10. A New Home?

My new home – professionally at least – was Rae, Bean and Partners. The practice is situated in the middle of Boroughbridge, exactly ten miles south of Thirsk. I knew the small town a little, from the time Anne had spent working there when we first came back up to Yorkshire. Now, though, I would be getting to know the historic town much more intimately.

In fact, the first ever time I came to the town was as a veterinary student, in 1991 or 1992. During our training, we had to do a spell of work experience at a veterinary laboratory. In those days, the government department that supervised disease control in farm animals was extensive. There was a network of Veterinary Investigation Centres (VICs) across the country whose role it was to monitor, diagnose, measure and report disease outbreaks in livestock. Thirsk had one of the biggest centres and my fellow trainee vet and friend Nick and I decided that this would be the best place to learn all about post-mortems on sheep, faeces-testing in cattle and disease control in poultry. Nick and I had been at school together in West Yorkshire and, by strange coincidence, both ended up studying veterinary medicine at Cambridge in the class of 1996. Nick's parents were caravan enthusiasts and kindly took their caravan to a site just outside Thirsk, so we had somewhere inexpensive to stay, close to the lab. For my part, I volunteered to drive my little red metro up the A1 to get us both there and to and from the VIC every day.

As we passed Boroughbridge, on the way to Thirsk, Nick suggested we stop for lunch. The Black Bull – an ancient pub, dating from the thirteenth century – was the obvious place for a pie and a pint. The pub is about the length of a cricket pitch from the practice in which I now work and I often think about that first visit, almost thirty years ago.

The fortnight at the VIC was interesting, or at least as interesting as working in a lab, chopping up dead and diseased animals, could be. Both Nick and I learnt plenty about post-mortem examinations, but the lack of contact with living patients and their owners was a frustration for me. On our last day, the senior veterinary surgeon presented us both with sealed envelopes containing his assessment of our training during the two-week block.

He insisted on seeing us both separately and made a big deal over the confidentiality of the report. This was a surprise, because most vets with whom we had seen practice would simply fill in the form and hand it straight back to us. The comments, whether positive or negative, would give us important feedback upon how we were progressing, helping us learn from our mistakes or identify areas of deficiency. A positive comment went a long way – encouragement was as important to a student then as it is now.

Anyhow, we both left the VIC and headed back to our caravan, clutching the all-important, sealed assessments – which we immediately opened. The secrecy of the palaver suggested there would be some serious comments about our performance.

Inside each envelope was written the same, disappointingly terse assessment: 'Satisfactory'

This was as deflating as it sounds. As a schoolboy, as a vet student, as a veterinary surgeon, or just in life, 'satisfactory' has never been something for which I have strived. There were no comments to suggest how I could improve from 'satisfactory' towards 'excellent', so the exercise in form-filling was rather pointless. But, it ticked a box I suppose, which was the essence of working for the State Veterinary Service.

That was a long time ago now. I hoped my professional life in Boroughbridge would be more than just 'satisfactory'.

The town has a lot of history and so has the veterinary surgery. Both justify a few pages in this book.

Boroughbridge is quintessentially English and, especially, quintessentially Yorkshire. The main street winds through the town with several sharp, right-angle bends. There are lots of pubs and a beautiful central square called St James Square, which has an iconic structure right in the middle, known as 'The Fountain'. Nobody knows why it is called this, because it's actually a well, and provided drinking water for the town until the 1930s. The square was the site for cattle sales in the early part of the twentieth century. The cattle market no longer exists but the middle of the town is still bustling, full of independent shops and small businesses. It is something of a local mantra that Boroughbridge has one of everything – a butcher, a baker and a candlestick maker, to quote the nursery rhyme. This isn't as far from the truth as you might think. There is still a butcher and a baker, and while there isn't a candlestick maker any more, candle-making was, in times past, an important industry for the town. The factory that made them functioned until 1937, sending candles to the shipyards of the north-east where they were used to illuminate ships' boilers.

The history of the town goes back way further than that, though. Standing in a field beside the A1 are three huge monoliths that go by the name of 'The Devil's Arrows'. These ancient stones are a sign that there was human activity in Boroughbridge as far back as 55 BC. The stones are made of millstone grit, originating from Plumpton Rocks, near Harrogate, some ten miles away. How, and perhaps more importantly, why they were moved here is enough to boggle the mind. The most likely theory is that they were waymarkers to indicate the route to the huge henge at Thornborough, further to the north. It seems an awful lot of effort to go to simply to make some signposts! I pass these monoliths every day and they never fail to impress me.

By the first century, the Romans had arrived in the town or, more specifically, the neighbouring village of Aldborough. In Roman times, this was a settlement called Isurium, an important stopping-off point on the road from York to Corbridge, near Hadrian's Wall. Travelling south from Aldborough towards York and beyond, it is still possible to see that the Romans had a hand in shaping the landscape; such is the directness of the route and the straightness of many of the roads.

In more recent history, the town thrived because of its strategic position, both for travel by road up and down the country and for transport of goods along the waterways. Wool from Nidderdale (particularly from Fountains Abbey) was taken overland to Boroughbridge, from where it could be loaded onto boats to take it down the River Ure to the Ouse, the Humber and out across the sea to Belgium, France and Italy. It's amazing to think, in these times of Brexit-fuelled xenophobia and insularity, that years ago trade between the heart of the Yorkshire Dales and continental Europe was driving the local economy! We should learn a lesson from our ancestors.

But, it was the Great North Road and the golden age of the

stagecoach, at the end of the Georgian era, that really put the town on the map. Just as the Romans had found it a perfect stopping-off point on their route to the north, so too did the traders and travellers who moved up and down the country by stagecoach.

One report, in a book called *A Picturesque History of Yorkshire 1899–1901*, recounts the bustling halcyon days of the stagecoach era in Boroughbridge perfectly:

> *Not only did the Great North Road pass through the town, but the bridge which carried it over the Ure was the only one between York and Ripon which was public to folk anxious to travel north or south. Consequently, the road was filled with a never-ceasing procession of wagons, packhorses, stagecoaches, post-chaises, droves of cattle, sheep, horses, private carriages and mail-coaches and all the heterogeneous life of eighteenth century road-side.*

Few of the coaching inns still remain, but it doesn't take much to imagine the life of a thriving town, its inns bursting with travellers, sweaty horses being watered and fed and the heady smells that accompany such activities. I've often wondered how many equine vets would have been required back then. Certainly, even as far back at the nineteenth century, veterinary surgeons were recorded as having practised in the town: John Lumley in 1829 and Joseph Thompson in 1841, with the fifteen-year-old William Faudle as his apprentice, followed by John Parke in the 1850s.

Given the rich history of the town, I should not have been surprised when I began to learn about the history of Rae, Bean and Partners. I had met both Alistair Rae and Vic Bean, although I did not know them well. Alistair retired from the practice soon after I started working in Thirsk in 1996, but he was very good friends with Jim Wight, the senior partner at Skeldale at that time– then it was called Sinclair and Wight (after Donald Sinclair and Alf Wight).

Jim and Alistair used to go on holiday together as children, long before their veterinary days. Both their fathers were veterinary surgeons. Alistair's father, Gordon Rae (who ran the practice before Alistair and Vic) was a great friend of Alf Wight, aka James Herriot. The story of how they met was serendipitous. Alf and his wife, Joan, would sometimes go for afternoon tea at Betty's Tea Rooms in Harrogate, to relax and escape the trials of farm-animal practice. So too would Gordon and his wife, Jean.

Gordon, hearing a familiar Scottish accent across the scones and jam and teapots, presumably speaking on an animal-related topic, went over to talk to Alf.

'Are you George Donaldson?' he asked, mistaking Alf for another Scottish veterinarian who had established (what became) a hugely successful mixed practice in West Yorkshire around the same time.

'I'm not. Why do you ask?' replied Alf.

'You look just like him. George and I were at school together in Strathallan,' Gordon explained.

'No. It's not me,' said Alf. 'The only person I know of from Strathallan is Gordon Rae, the vet at Boroughbridge.'

'That's funny,' replied Gordon, '*I'm* Gordon Rae from Boroughbridge vets. Pleased to meet you!'

And so began a lifelong friendship between the two vets. They met up nearly every Thursday afternoon in Harrogate and worked just down the road from each other. As Jim Wight recalled in his biography of his father, *The Real James Herriot*, Gordon and Alf were

both slaves to general practice and had many an amusing
tale to tell. It was an especial comfort to Alf, as he laughed
at Gordon's stories of triumph and catastrophe, that his
exacting life as a veterinary surgeon was one that was shared
by so many of his colleagues. Alf would never tire of the
company of Gordon Rae.

The work at Alf's surgery in Thirsk and Gordon Rae's practice
in Boroughbridge was very similar. They both covered huge
distances to treat farm animals across Yorkshire. Alf looked after
a multitude of farms as far as Wensleydale, carrying out TB-
testing for hundreds of small herds. At Skeldale, my old home,
there was an enormous collection of worn, old and stained
notebooks, each with the scrawled handwriting of Alf or Donald
Sinclair, with ear-tag numbers and skin-test readings taken from
cattle from all over the north of the county. Similarly, at the
Boroughbridge surgery, in an old and yellowing daybook there
is a record of a visit to see a pig in Brough, some sixty miles
away, in the wilds of Westmorland. The visit cost five shillings
and the pig received a bottle of lotion for its sore skin.

Both Gordon and Alf, as we've discovered, had sons who
followed their fathers into the veterinary profession. When the
time came for the two men to retire, Alistair Rae took over from
his father at Boroughbridge, while Jim Wight took charge at
Thirsk. Alistair was soon joined at Boroughbridge by his friend,
Vic Bean. Vic and Alistair had been at university together, and
had also worked together at another veterinary practice, well
known at the time, in Penkridge, Staffordshire. This was the
home of a veterinary surgeon called Eddie Straiton, with whom,
coincidentally, Jim had also worked at the start of his veterinary
career. Rumour has it that Eddie could spay a cat in under five
minutes and could complete hundreds of visits each week, racing

around the Staffordshire countryside in his open-topped sports car. Eddie removed his shirt at every opportunity, too. Even (apparently) to spay a cat.

The story goes that, on the evening of Vic's first date with his future wife, Gina, he was late, tied up calving a cow. He sent his friend Alistair to Gina's house to collect her and drop her off at the farm. To me, this plan was flawed – even if everything had gone smoothly, a vet who had just finished a calving would have been dirty, smelly and slimy and in no fit state for a date with a new girlfriend. However, only slightly anxious, Gina, dressed in the latest Mary Quant, clambered into Alistair's tatty car and they headed through the dark and winding lanes of Staffordshire to find Vic, who was up to his shoulders in cow. Eddie was there too, to help the young vet. According to Gina, the moment she stepped out of the car, carefully avoiding mud, Eddie ceremoniously stripped off his shirt, as if to emphasise his position as alpha male.

Eddie also appeared on *The Jimmy Young Show* offering veterinary advice. He was known as 'The TV vet' and wrote several books. I would urge anyone with an interest in veterinary literature to track some of these books down. My particular favourite is one called *Cats: Their Health and Care*. There is a fantastic picture of Eddie demonstrating how to revive a cat that you have rescued from drowning, by holding its back legs and swinging the poor creature above his head – I'm sure, again, without his shirt. If you look carefully, there is a wide-eyed, staring look about the cat that suggests rigor mortis had long since set in. The image could have come straight out of a Monty Python episode.

Vic and Alistair had always planned to run their own practice, so when the opportunity arose in Boroughbridge, Vic left Staffordshire to join his friend. He was a wonderful vet, compassionate and practical at the same time. He became an expert on pigs and I remember having a long conversation with him in the car park of the Veterinary Investigation Centre in Thirsk one day. I was dropping off a faeces sample and a vial of blood from a patient and Vic was probably taking a pig for a post-mortem. It was not long after I'd started in Thirsk and, even though I was clearly a novice in the profession and he was a master, he spent twenty minutes out of his busy day chatting to me, discussing interesting cases that he had on the go, as well as various bits of gossip from the veterinary and farming world. He was a kind man and someone whom everyone admired.

So, Rae, Bean and Partners had a long history and a proud heritage, very much in the Herriot tradition. As I delved a bit deeper, I discovered that, even before Gordon Rae's time, there were stories aplenty!

There is a record of a veterinary surgeon called Thomas Secker, who practised in the town in 1902. The surgery at that time was down by the River Ure. Thomas had a terrible accident while making a horse medicine out of chlorate of potash, sulphur and iron. Goodness knows what effect the medicine would have had on the horse, but there was a huge explosion in the veterinary practice, which blew out all of the windows and smashed all of the furniture. It also blew off the vet's arm and part of his leg, which then apparently had to be amputated – on his own operating table – in an attempt to save him. But the attempt was unsuccessful, and the poor man subsequently died as a result of his injuries. This story took me back to my childhood, when I too created a similarly explosive mixture in my parents' greenhouse. I must have been about ten when I decided to make some gunpowder. Luckily for me, my concoction only blew out one pane of glass and no body parts were lost. I hoped my career as a vet in Boroughbridge would be more successful than that of Mr Secker.

Following the explosion (in the Boroughbridge vets', not my parents' greenhouse), the practice was taken over by William Campbell, who was followed by Gordon Rae in 1942. In those days, the vet lived as well as worked at the practice. In his first attempt to tidy up the house, Gordon set about some renovations, including opening up a bricked-up fireplace. Much to his surprise, as he moved some of the stones the well-preserved, blown-off arm of the aforementioned Mr Secker fell out, amongst the soot. It was still clutching his pipe!

Everyone I met in Boroughbridge, both small-animal clients and farmers alike, immediately made me very welcome. So, although moving practices was a huge upheaval for me, I couldn't have had it any easier.

One farmer called me out to see a cow at a lovely farm in Aldborough, just down the road from the practice, on a day when the wind was blowing cold from the north and a biting sleet was falling. The cow had recently calved and had not yet passed her placenta. She needed cleansing. This is a simple but smelly procedure, requiring no particular veterinary skill or experience, just sufficient layers of plastic gloves to avoid the fetid stench permeating through to the skin of the arms and hands, where it lingers indelibly for days.

The cow, a huge, docile British Blue cross, was penned up in the corner of the fold yard, behind a gate and out of the wintery weather. Her calf stood by, oblivious to the smelly membranes hanging from its mother's back end.

'I'm glad it's you that's come, Julian,' said the farmer, shaking my hand. 'I heard you'd come to this practice and I've heard a lot about you. I thought it'd be good to meet you, to make your acquaintance, like.'

He continued, 'it's a good thing you've come to this practice, yer know. It needed a man like you. I hope you'll stick around.'

It was a ringing endorsement before I'd actually had the opportunity to demonstrate my skills. I just hoped I would live up to the expectations of the clients and that I could do justice to this historic practice. It was quickly becoming clear to me that it was a practice more Herriot than Herriot and that its ethos sat comfortably with my own. Would this be my permanent veterinary home? It was too early to tell but time and circumstances would provide the answer, I felt sure.

11. The Yorkshire Vet Continues

I pulled on my new woolly hat before I arrived at the farm, trying to trap some of the warmth from my car. The wind was buffeting the bare trees, whose roots strained to stay attached to the ground. It wasn't even particularly high up where I was heading – the small sheep farm near Marton cum Grafton had an elevated position, with views over the Vale of York and towards the Wolds, but it could hardly be compared to the wilds of Dallowgill, on the edge of Nidderdale, nor to the bleak Hambleton Hills that I had frequented in the past. Nevertheless, I knew my next call would be a cold affair. I hadn't been to the farm before but I had been to their neighbours – that had been a bleak episode too – so I knew approximately where I was going. The patient awaiting my attention today was a ewe, struggling to lamb.

'There's a lambing just come in. It's a head out.' Julie, the nurse, had pushed a scrap of paper into my hand with the farmer's name and address, within just a few minutes of my return to the surgery from another call. 'It's next to Grass Hills where you went the other week to see that bullock.' Julie was well aware that this was no time for discussion or detailed instructions. A lamb with just its head out was a veterinary emergency. I jumped straight back into the car and reached for my hat. My recent visit to the next-door farm had also seen me grappling with something hanging from a farm animal's back end, but on that occasion it was a bullock with a prolapsed rectum, outside in a squally shower of sleet and rain. Although it had been bitterly cold, the bullock was fine, and I hoped this visit to the gentle, hanging valley would have just as happy an outcome.

I drove past Grass Hills and upwards across a wooded hillside looking for my destination in the approaching gloom of a January late afternoon. But it was easy to find – at the next bend, Woodlands Farm was right in front of me. I pulled up in front of a large barn door, through which I could see lines of Texel sheep, hungrily munching on hay. I knew I was in the right place and got out to find the farmer.

'Oh, hello. She's in there,' came a voice. An elderly lady, bent double over a ski-pole-like stick, was making her way across the yard towards the farmhouse, picking her way carefully around the patches of frozen mud. 'I'll get Bill.'

'Bill! It's the vet,' she bellowed, much more loudly than I would have expected from her diminutive figure. Bill appeared at the back door.

I introduced myself.

'Hello, I'm Julian. I gather you've got problems with a sheep?'

'Yes, she has a head out,' confirmed Bill. 'Both legs back. I knew it'd be too much for me so I called you straight away. It only makes it worse if a farmer messes around when it's a job for the vet. And, by the way, I do know who you are: I've seen you on the telly. M' wife and I watch you every Tuesday. We think it's great.'

Bill was anxious about his ewe, but his eyes smiled, maybe because he was pleased to meet me, maybe because he was confident I could help, or maybe because I was the first person the old farmer had ever met in real life who he'd seen on television.

I smiled too, concurring with his comments.

'Yes, you're right. It's a serious business if the head's out, but I'll do my best. Have you got a bucket of water please?' And then, to acknowledge his comments about being on telly, I simply added, 'It is a bit strange, I have to admit!'

I could hear Bill and his wife from outside the farmhouse as they grappled with a large bucket of water from the kitchen.

'Can you manage it?' asked his frail wife, as the elderly farmer, just as hunched but without a stick, hobbled out of the house with the bucket, which I quickly took off his hands, and an off-white towel. I wasn't quite sure what she would have done if he'd replied saying he couldn't manage.

I followed him into the barn, where the ewe had been penned. She wasn't happy about being confined in a small space and was perturbed both by the presence of a stranger and the strange sensation at her back end of the lamb's swollen head. She ran around and around in the straw-filled pen, making it hard for Bill to catch her. I put the bucket of precious warm water safely to one side and lent a hand, concerned for the farmer and for the future of the partly born lamb. I'd seen sheep in similar situations before, charging around a field with a lamb's head bouncing about violently, the rest of its body stuck in the birth canal and it didn't usually end well. Anyhow, with two of us working together, the ewe was soon captured and standing in position, the bucket of water was in place and I could make a start. The low barn had no lights, and very little natural light managed to filter through the gaps, so it was actually very hard to see the sheep, the farmer or the lamb's head. Luckily, this didn't really matter as I could work just by feel. Anything more involved, like a Caesarean, would have necessitated rummaging around for head-torches and lamps, but for now I ploughed on in the semi-darkness.

For a normal delivery, it is preferable for the lamb to be presented with the two front legs coming first, closely followed by the head, positioned like a swimmer diving into a pool. A lamb can be delivered without assistance if the back legs come first, and, occasionally (for example, if the lamb is small or the ewe capacious) with a head and just one front leg pointing forward. If both front legs are folded back and just a head has appeared, then without intervention the lamb will die quickly; its blood supply will constrict, causing the head to swell dangerously. With plenty of lubrication, and sometimes also with an epidural injection to numb the area and prevent the ewe from pushing, the head can be gently pushed back inside to allow manipulation of the front legs into alignment so that the lamb can be born. In this case, the head was very swollen and not at all easy to get back into the birth canal. I knew it would take me a while, so as I worked on coaxing the lamb into position, I chatted to Bill about his flock and his farm.

'I have forty this year to lamb, so it's not that many I suppose,' he explained with a broad Yorkshire accent and equally broad grin. 'Abart half as many as last year, I'm getting awd and every year I keep a few less. It's not so easy nowadays.'

Then, 'This is my first sheep to lamb this year – a vet visit to the first lambing isn't a very good start – I hope I don't need you for every one of them!'

I was making progress and, thankfully, I soon had the head back inside. After that, it wasn't too hard to get the legs up to join the head and before long Bill's first lamb of the season was lying in deep straw, with the ewe licking it vigorously. It had been a success and I'd made a new acquaintance. Bill, however, seemed to feel as if he knew me very well already. After all, *he'd seen me on telly*.

'I feel like I know you, Julian. I've seen you on telly,' was a phrase I heard very frequently in the first few weeks and months in my new practice – more than once every day, in fact. It was a peculiar experience, to add to the variety of other peculiar experiences that I had accumulated over the last couple of years. Starting a new job always involves meeting new people and settling in. You must establish your veterinary credentials and convince the clients that you know what you're doing. This process can take many months – at least until the less satisfactory outcomes are outweighed by the successes, like Bill's lambing, for example. You need to persuade a farmer that you *do* know how to calve a cow, and give confidence to a worried cat owner that, 'yes, I have done this operation plenty of times before and it really is very safe and definitely the best thing for Felix.' But, I didn't have to do this at all. The majority of the pet- and farm-animal-owning public in Yorkshire were well acquainted with the TV programme, and even those who weren't had often read my column in the *Yorkshire Post*, so, in a rather disarming way, my reputation (or if not my actual reputation, certainly my existence as someone people recognised) preceded me. It made it easier and it made it harder and it made it interesting, all at the same time. It took some getting used to, that's for sure.

I thought that the sale of James Herriot's former practice to a huge corporate chain, with mainly small-animal interests, would spell the end of *The Yorkshire Vet*. By the time I left Skeldale, we had made well over fifty episodes. It had been hard work, but a lot of fun and a wonderful opportunity that I had never expected to have. There was always an element of anxiety associated with exposing yourself and your practice to the TV-viewing public, putting yourself completely on display and under scrutiny. But the rewards of being able to share the joy of delivering a lamb with two million people made it all worthwhile. The lovely comments from fans and the warm letters of appreciation by far outweighed the occasional unpleasant social media comment criticising a clinical approach or the handling of a case. It had been an interesting and an exciting time, but I was a veterinary surgeon and not a television presenter, and my intention was to continue in my vocation as a mixed practitioner. At Channel 5, however, there was clearly a desire to continue with the programme – commissioning editors don't give up their high-rating shows just like that. I was still working in Yorkshire, albeit in a different practice, so, from their point of view, there was still ample scope to continue my involvement. I would, after all (in the words of the opening sequence to the programme), still be 'Continuing the Herriot tradition, treating All Creatures Great and Small'. So, the inevitable question came: Would I like to carry on with *The Yorkshire Vet*?

It took some serious thought. Did I want to share my (by now quite public) move from my (now famous) previous practice with everyone who watched *The Yorkshire Vet*? It would put me under the spotlight even more than before, which would not be easy. On the other hand, in the context of the big changes facing me, the one constant would be to continue filming, and at the very least I'd get to carry on working with the camera crews and production teams who had become my friends over the preceding three years. In the end, it was a fairly easy decision and I agreed to continue the filming. The start of a new chapter in my veterinary career, challenging as it would undoubtedly be, would be caught on camera for the animal-loving population of the UK to share.

One of the first cases I saw at Boroughbridge, and I think the very first one to be filmed, was Tom and his cockerel. I'd seen his name on the appointment list, and also the problem with his favourite bird, when I'd checked the previous day. I picked up the phone:

'Laura, will you be in tomorrow?' I asked my trusty producer-director. 'I've got a farmer coming in. He thinks there's a boil on his cock!'

I knew what her answer would be.

Lo and behold, Laura was already in position with her camera when I arrived at work the following morning to see Tom about the problem with his cock. There was not a trace of innuendo. Promise.

The problem was a genuine one and Tom, the tall, broad-shouldered young farmer with rugged Buzz Lightyear good looks, was genuinely worried about his favourite cockerel. And the cockerel did actually have a boil – well, a nasty infected swelling, at least. It was on the underside of his neck. It had appeared suddenly and was bleeding and ulcerated. Moreover, both he and his harem of hens were giving it their full attention with their beaks, which was only making matters worse. The boil needed some fairly urgent attention, but alongside that Laura and I were both well aware that Tom and his cockerel had all the ingredients of a super story for the TV.

'Tom, I think the only thing I can do is to remove it,' I said gravely. Even though Laura had painstakingly avoided all innuendo, there was no hiding it now, and although the situation was quite serious, we all started to laugh.

'I'm just glad you can help, Julian.' Tom sounded relieved.

'You'll probably think I'm a big, daft softie, but I love this bird and I just want him right. I know you'll do a good job. Thank you for helping.'

Tom seemed to have confidence in my ability, even though this was the first time we had met. He'd seen me on telly too.

I gathered up the bird in its basket. 'See ya, Neil,' Tom called as he headed out of the practice to await my phone call, telling him how the procedure had gone. Yes, the cockerel was called Neil!

I took Neil-the-cockerel to the kennels, looking for a volunteer from the nursing staff to assist me. Again, Julie came to the rescue and offered to help. She had not anaesthetised a cockerel before. Neither had she ever been filmed for television. Laura and I tried to offer her some reassurance.

'Just be normal,' I said. 'It's easy. Just do what you do. Don't worry and relax.'

She didn't look convinced, given the dual challenge of coping with the camera and putting a huge cockerel under anaesthetic. I had done both these things before, so I hoped that if I was calm about it, Julie would be too. This worked – up to a point: the point at which Neil decided to flap his mighty wings and escape from the operating table just as we were hooking him up to the gas. Chaos ensued for a few moments, but Julie quickly managed to gather the bird back up and we all regained some composure. From then on, everything went very smoothly. It turned out to be a relatively minor op, and Neil was soon recovering in a kennel.

I called Tom to pass on the news that the surgery had been successful and that his bird had recovered uneventfully from the anaesthetic. He was delighted and I could hear the relief in his voice down the phone. However, later in the day as we got Neil ready to go home, Julie spotted a potential problem.

'Is he going to peck at his wound, Julian?'

The naughty cockerel had, prior to his arrival at the practice, already been pecking at the boil, so he was certain to do the same to the sutures. We needed to find a way to prevent him from doing this. Normally we would use some sort of collar – buster collars, Elizabethan collars, lampshades, satellite dishes, call them what you will – which are all designed to prevent animals interfering with their sutures or making wounds worse. I'd never used one on a bird though, so the next ten minutes were quite an experience as we experimented with plastic collars of various shapes and sizes. Neil looked more and more dejected with every new style we tried around his neck. I'd never realised a cockerel could look so sad.

Then, Julie had an inspired idea. We had some different collars that, instead of being made of hard plastic, were inflatable rubber armbands, just like the ones toddlers wear to keep them afloat in a swimming pool. A collar like this is supposed to stop a dog from being able to bend its neck round to reach a row of stitches somewhere further back on its body. This would be more comfortable for Neil. Minutes later, I'd blown up the rubber ring and we fastened it around the cockerel's neck with the Velcro straps provided. Well, either the ring was too heavy, or Neil was still weak from his recent anaesthetic, or it was a combination of the two, but the effect was like putting heavy wellington boots onto a duck (not that this is something I've ever done either). The poor bird's head drooped forward so that his beak rested on the table, and there he stayed, dejected, surprised and a bit sad.

'Well,' I said, 'at least he'll stay afloat if he falls in the duck pond!'

It was clearly not going to be a feasible way of protecting the stitches and we decided we would just have to cross our fingers and hope he wouldn't peck the wound too much. He went home later that afternoon. As I reunited Tom with his bird and bade them both farewell, I was sure there was a small tear in the corner of the farmer's eye. I couldn't tell for sure whether it was a tear of emotion or a tear of laughter from seeing his beloved cockerel with a rubber ring around his neck, but I think I knew!

12. Gilbert the Micro-Pig

I got to know Tom and his family very well over the following few months. Winter was beginning to relax its grip on North Yorkshire and I paid their farm several visits, attending to more conventional veterinary tasks, as the snow began to thaw. I checked Neil the cockerel every time. He made a spectacular recovery from his ordeal.

The first time I met Tom's father, Richard, he looked familiar. His mannerisms, his voice and his obvious love of his animals reminded me of another farmer, called John, with whom I'd worked back in Thirsk. I'd spent many long days castrating and dehorning John's wonderful prize-winning cattle, avoiding well-aimed kicks for hours at a time. John would use old carpets to line the sides on the cattle crush to make it easier on his cattle, and he would put his old hockey shin pads inside his wellies to make it easier on his own lower limbs, just in case the kicks strayed in his direction. It turned out that John and Richard were brothers, with a resemblance so striking they could have been twins. I'd lambed countless sheep for John, usually, as I recall, in the small hours of the morning or on Sundays in spring. And as for the almost daily visits to calve cows during the famous winter of 2009, when the whole country was overtaken by arctic weather, well that's another story altogether . . .

So, Richard was someone else who felt he knew me very well, even before we'd met. Not just because of the family connection, and also, for once, not because of the TV, but on account of my books, which he had enjoyed (luckily). At least on this occasion, by virtue of knowing Richard's brother, I could claim some sort of reciprocity.

Their farm was a traditional Yorkshire set-up. It was very mixed, operating a small flock of sheep, alongside a suckler herd of handsome Limousin cattle, each of which had a story and each of which held a special place in the heart of this kind farming family. They also had a belligerent Jack Russell terrier, who was always locked in the tractor when I arrived, to avoid confrontation. And, of course, they had a few hens.

My first visit was to dehorn a bunch of heifers – a necessary but not very appealing job – and that was followed by a smattering of lambings and the treatment of a few poorly sheep during lambing time. I started to feel that I had justified my place as their vet by good jobs done, rather than by a reputation that preceded me, and this made me happy. But there was one case I was having trouble fixing – an old cow with a bad foot. She had calved recently, and infection had taken hold in her back foot. It was painful and swollen and had stubbornly refused to improve despite the usual injections. It was disappointing for all concerned, especially the cow, and I felt like my hard-earned position of respect was on a knife-edge. I agreed to have another look, one last try.

'Richard, I think the only thing I can do now is to amputate this claw,' I declared, bravely. This was not a widely used procedure and I expected some face-pulling from the wise and experienced farmer.

'Well, I have heard about that sort of thing in the past.' Richard nodded. 'I think Vic might have talked about it once or twice before.' I had quickly come to realise that when farmers around Boroughbridge spoke about something that Vic had once done, it meant they thought everything would be all right. I have never heard more people in an area speak in unison with so much respect for one man. So, even though this would be a difficult procedure and one with no guarantee of success, if Vic had mentioned it, I would have no problem persuading Richard that it was the right course of action. I arranged to come back the following day to carry out the operation.

The infection was affecting one of the digits on the cow's back foot. Cows, like sheep, pigs and deer, have two claws on each foot. This is different from a horse, where the lower part of the leg has developed into a single hoof, or from a dog or cat where there are five digits on the front legs but usually only four on the back. It was another example of the *comparative anatomy* that we'd studied at vet school. I was never very good at anatomy – too many complicated words to memorise – but I was always fascinated by the anatomical differences between different species and how and why they developed as they did. These different leg arrangements are all to do with adaptations for running fast. Carnivores are light and nimble, whereas herbivores, which are heavier because of the huge gut they require to digest grass, get their speed by having longer, stronger legs.

Cows bear most of the weight of the back half of their body on the outside claw of each back foot, so if lameness develops in the foot it almost always originates from the outside digit. This was indeed the case in Richard's cow. The infection in the poor cow's foot was well established and had invaded all the important structures – the bone, the flexor tendons and, I thought, also the joint. I explained it all to Richard, who was keen to give it a go.

'Well, put it this way, Julian,' said Richard, 'we ain't got a lot to lose 'ave we? She's in an awful lot of pain, the injections haven't worked and I'd like her to have the rest of the year ahead so she can rear her calf. She's an old cow, but she's been a good 'un and I'd like to give it a go. If you think there's a chance I'd like to try.'

Richard's endorsement of my plan was not exactly ringing. He was pragmatic enough to realise that the ambitious op might not work.

I set about the task with a degree of trepidation. It was some years since I had last carried out such a procedure. It was something I had performed fairly frequently in the early part of my career – the good old days of dairy farming, when dairy cows were very precious and milk was valuable. Milking cows needed to be fit and pain-free, and a vet would not infrequently be called on to amputate a claw to save a good milker. Sadly, for reasons that are hard to rationalise, milk prices have been terrible over recent decades. The economics of this type of farming now dictate that a lame dairy cow is put out of its pain in a more final way, rather than go through this fairly involved surgery. It is not a good thing, in my opinion, but unfortunately this is the way it is. Modern dairy cows do not, generally, enjoy the same long and healthy lives as beef suckler cows, which is a shame.

Richard's cow, therefore, was lucky she wasn't a dairy cow. Richard cared deeply for his animals and wanted to give the old girl a chance. With her leg held up by a rope, I applied a tourniquet near to her hock. This served two purposes – to reduce any bleeding that might occur during the surgery, and also to allow me to inject a big syringe of local anaesthetic into a prominent vein in the lower limb. This is a technique called 'intravenous regional anaesthesia' and it is very useful. When performed correctly, it renders the whole of the lower limb completely numb, allowing any type of surgical intervention. Today, the surgical intervention was very basic. I would be sawing off half of the cow's foot – the bit with the infection eating away at the joint and the bone. I used special wire, which we would usually use to cut off horns in young cattle and is similar to the wire a delicatessen would use to slice cheese. It was not fancy or glamorous and it was definitely not something you'd see on an episode of *The Supervet*, but it was mightily effective; within just a few moments, the bad bit of foot was off. I applied a thick bandage, administered more drugs to keep the discomfort at bay and gently lowered the remaining healthy digit to the ground. Then came the moment of truth. As soon as we let the cow out of the crush, her calf came running up to her side and miraculously, for the first time in weeks, the conker-coloured cow put some pressure on her back right leg. So far, so good!

'By gum, that's a good job,' said Richard.

I felt quite pleased, too. Provided everything healed up nicely, the cow was, at least for the foreseeable future, saved. As I cleaned my wellies, climbed into the car and drove off down the long farm lane, I couldn't help feeling that Vic would have been proud!

Not long after my op on Richard's cow, I was presented with another painful foot to treat, this time belonging to an enormous Clydesdale horse. Howard had ongoing problems with his dinner-plate-sized hooves and his huge left front foot was sore again. Several previous vets had been struggling to keep him right and now it was my turn.

'I'd love it if you could come and have a look at Howard,' said

Collette, his owner, on the phone. 'It's his foot again. He's just standing in the field. I can't ride him, you see, at the moment, but when he does walk it's definitely giving him some pain.'

'I'd also like you to meet Gilbert,' she added. 'Gilbert doesn't have anything wrong with him at the moment. But I love him so much. He's a micro-pig.'

Already, my mind was filling with images of enormous horses and tiny pigs, cohabiting in some sort of rural idyll.

It took a bit of juggling to work out a suitable time to visit Collette and her menagerie. This sunny springtime was busier than any other I had known. Two vets were out of action and in hospital, leaving those still standing overworked and struggling to fit in even the routine cases. Eventually I found half a morning to put aside to see Collette, her enormous horse and her micro-pig. Her directions were spot on and I easily found the field. It had so many buttercups flowering in it that it was more yellow than it was green, but nevertheless I could tell even before I met the animals that this was a beautiful home for pigs and horses of any shape or size.

Collette greeted me like a long-lost friend, immediately intro-ducing me to the lame Clydesdale after the faithful old boy had hobbled up to me, his enormous head nodding rhythmically each time his right foot touched the ground and bobbing up each time his left fore took the weight. Moving much more quickly, clearly preoccupied with pig-thoughts and almost hidden by the tall buttercups, was Gilbert. He was hardly the micro-pig I'd imagined; he took up as much space as any standard-sized pig. Even the micro-pigs were huge on this farm!

'And this is my little Gilbert.' Collette smiled. 'I love this little pig. He's my soulmate.'

But it was Howard who needed my attention. I held out my hand for him to nuzzle as I tried to work out how to lift the huge foot and start my examination. It was heavy and, although Howard was very gentle, he did not like me picking it up at all. Once I started paring at the rock-hard sole with my hoof knives, exploring the fissures and small cracks that might lead me to the pocket of black pus that was causing the pain, the giant stomped his foot down, stubbornly refusing to make my job even possible, let alone easy. Eventually, with much sweating, backache and some persuasion, I managed to work out a system of paring away a few slivers of sole at a time, leading me slowly towards the affected area. Just as I felt I was winning, Gilbert emerged from the buttercups, snuffling along to see what I was up to. He'd come to say 'hello', but quickly became very interested in both my shoelaces and, more critically, my hoof knives and hoof testers. Once he had untied my shoelaces, he set about removing the all-important knives, skipping as he carried them off in his mouth. His charm was endearing, but it was certainly not helping me treat Howard's foot.

'Naughty Howard!' I kept hearing myself say as the enormous horse stomped his foot down again.

'Naughty Gilbert!' I'd call to the pig as he chugged off into the buttercups with my equipment.

Collette was helping to retrieve the things I needed, but it was a fruitless task and in the end she resorted to distracting the pig with a small tub of ice cream.

'Gilbert loves an ice cream, especially on a hot day like today,' she explained as the pig stuffed his snout into the small plastic pot. It was a perfect distraction, although after half an hour of sweating with a heavy horse's foot, I was longing for an ice cream myself! Eventually, though, my work was done – a bluish-black trickle of pus exuded from a hole I'd dug in the sole, next to the hoof wall. It was a classic case. The infection had become trapped, resulting in a painful build-up of pressure inside the unyielding tissues of the hoof. I was relieved to find the source, although in reality I was not convinced this was the full story. The problems were deep-seated and Howard's feet were suffering from structural changes that led me to suspect this might not be the last time I would be grappling with his feet.

I wiped the sweat from my eyes and straightened out my wrecked back, wondering how on earth farriers coped with this many times a day.

I talked through the aftercare with Collette, explaining about poulticing and soaking the foot in warm, strong salt water to soften the sole and draw out any more pockets of infection.

'And now, Julian,' she declared, 'I've got an ice cream for *you*, too. You deserve it! I'm so pleased you could do something for Howard, and glad you've met my lovely little pig.' Collette reached into her coolbox and produced an ice cream for me and then for herself. We sat on a fence, enjoying the sunshine, and watched as the pig and the horse sauntered into the field. Collette told me the stories of how she came to have both the little pig (when he was actually little) and Howard, and described some of their funny habits: how Gilbert loved to sit in a paddling pool when it was hot; how he followed Howard everywhere and how he and Collette had a very special relationship. Finally, with a flourish and a hint of embarrassment, Collette pulled a piece of paper from her pocket.

'I've written a poem about Gilbert. Would you like to hear it?'

Well, this was the first and actually the only time I'd been invited to be the audience for a poetry recital about an animal, especially one read by the author and about the pig standing at my feet with ice cream on his snout. It seemed rude not to sit back and enjoy the sunshine, my ice cream, the view, the company and the poem. It went like this:

Hi, my name is Gilbert
I'm a piglet not quite a year old,
I never ever get told off
Because I'm truly as good as gold.

My breed is a 'micro-pig'
But my mum doesn't think so,
Because all I seem to do is grow
And grow and grow.

I'm all pink and wrinkly
And still my mum loves me,
Of that there is no doubt
I love it when she kisses me
On my mucky flat snout
Hey, and that's when I've had a right good root about!

My mum's called Collette,
She says: 'Who's Mummy's pet?'
I only have to cough or sneeze
And she'll go and call the vet.

Boy, does she look after me,
I get breakfast, lunch and tea,
There's also lots of snacks.
Mum says: 'Gilbert you're getting rather fat!'
Oh, I hope she doesn't think about
Cutting those cream cakes back!

We have lots of fun, me and Mum,
She tickles my tum and scratches my bum,
And lets me out to play,

I nibble on grass, pig nuts and hay,
To makes sure I'm safe
She puts me in at the end of the day.

She strokes my head as I'm laid
Snug in my bed.
That's made of thick, fresh straw,
Now tell me what more
Could a little piggy ask for?

I've no need to fear as
My mum is here,
And nor should I ever fret,
Am I a happy little piggy? You bet!
Oh, how I love being my mummy's pet!

Collette bent forward and patted Gilbert on his ice-creamy nose.

'Well done, Gilbert, my love. That's your poem, that is! Isn't it a lovely one! You're my favourite little piggy!'

I clapped with gusto. What an amazing thing. I'd quickly realised the strength of the bond between Collette and her animals, especially Gilbert. I sincerely hoped he would never be poorly. The weight of responsibility would be too much to bear!

In modern pig-farming, veterinary care is usually provided by specialist pig vets, of whom there are only a few. Large-scale production means that a handful of veterinary surgeons are responsible for treating huge herds spread across large swathes of the country. Individual pig care is not as common as it was in the days of my predecessors, when there was a pig in a pen at the end of every backyard. That said, the popularity of pigs such as Gilbert – micro-pigs, Kunekune pigs, Vietnamese

Pot-bellied ones and so on – has brought these fascinating creatures back onto the visit list of most mixed practitioners over recent years, as has the re-emergence of rare-breed pig-rearing, as farmers look for ways to diversify and move away from intensive methods. Difficult to handle as they can sometimes be, a pig certainly adds a lot of extra interest to a day otherwise filled with cows, sheep, dogs and cats. They are lovely to treat and their mischievous habits lead to all sorts of funny stories. I have a friend, who must remain nameless for reasons that will become clear, who often sends me amusing anecdotes about the pigs and their antics on her farm.

She sent me a funny story describing her and her husband Tom's first attempts to artificially inseminate a sow, when he accidentally inserted the catheter into the wrong orifice and tried to squirt the precious, imported semen up the sow's anus! A few months later, another ping in my inbox related yet another piece of comedy from their pig farm on the moors.

Hi Julian,
I hope you're keeping well. I thought I'd give you a giggle.

I hand-reared a piglet in May and called him Johnny. He's six months old now.

I hadn't the heart to have him castrated as he's my baby. He doesn't think he's a pig. He follows me around like a dog. I've taught him some tricks, he can sit, walk by my side and he does weave through plastic fence posts like an agility dog. Now, he is so spoilt he will only eat if he's hand-fed, plus his hormones have now kicked in, causing problems for Tom when he comes near me.

A couple of weeks ago a friend came to visit, who

had a false leg. I had Johnny out on a walk and, when we returned, he was surprised to see a stranger on the farm. Johnny welcomed him and wagged his tail and grunted happily. Suddenly, all hell broke loose, as the guy's false leg squeaked at the knee. Johnny didn't like it.

He started attacking the false leg, aiming at the squeaking knee joint. Our friend tried to walk away, but Johnny just held on, now shaking it with his teeth. Eventually he managed to break free, but Johnny went in again, headbutting the squeaking limb and then seizing it with his jaws again. Eventually I managed to call off the pig, but the poor chap's trousers were sodden with boar froth from his mouth!

I was laughing my head off, but thought I'd never see my friend again. But he came back again last week, to help out when my Tom was in hospital for a day. Funnily enough, another pig went for his squeaky limb – I told him he needs to get some oil on it. He said I should keep my pigs under control!

So, no harm was done and everyone remained friends (except perhaps Johnny and his nemesis with the squeaky leg). Johnny was clearly another pig with a strong bond with his owner. Not one who snuffled in the buttercups, stealing hoof knives and eating ice cream, but one who went for walks on a lead and did dog tricks. Both had prompted their owners to put their antics down on paper. Troublesome as they can be, I wish I got to see more pigs, because I love them a little bit too!

13. Old Friends and an Injured Cat

The sun was beating down relentlessly as I pulled on my wellies and waterproof trousers. These were not ideal clothes to be wearing in a heatwave and I was not relishing the next hour or so. Mr Wilkins had given me perfect directions to the farm, which he and his brother had been running for more decades than either of them could remember. A satnav would have been no use to me, I thought, as I followed the tiny lanes that wound steeply up and down, through long-dried-up fords and across large, open expanses of moorland. The heather-clad moors of North Yorkshire look their resplendent best in the middle of August when their tops wear a blanket of regal purple, and today they were more colourful than ever as I wound my way across and through them.

The purpose of my visit was to TB-test some cattle who had recently arrived on the farm. It was a task that gave James Herriot the opportunity to travel across the self-same moors when he was a young vet and was part of the inspiration for his famous books. The two brothers I was seeing today could have been straight out of one of his stories.

As I introduced myself to the elderly farmers, sweat was already beginning to form on my plastic-clad body.

'Good morning! It's a nice day for it!' I offered.

'Aye. It's a bit warm,' came the truculent reply from one Mr Wilkins.

The two old boys, surely into their eighties, moved slowly. They had made some concessions to the heat. Jackets and ties – the uniform for farmers from this era – had been discarded. So too had the flat caps. Even overalls had been rolled down to the waist. A casual look, if there was such a thing, for the pair of octogenarian brothers. As I clambered over the gate into the collecting pen, I noticed that both farmers had their gloves shoved into a back pocket, just in case the weather turned. There was zero chance of this, with not a cloud in the sapphire sky. There hadn't been a cloud in the sky for about two weeks and during this prolonged heatwave the temperature had been rising day by day. The grass was wilting and taking on a shade more like hay than its typical green, and there wasn't a lot of it. Grass needs plenty of water to grow and the drought was leaving reservoirs low and grazing cattle hungry. However, the thirty or so black and white Friesians who were my patients today looked anything but hungry. These old farmers knew exactly how to manage their cattle in all weathers, be it blizzards or drought, and the animals were all in great condition, with glossy coats and bright, inquisitive eyes.

I needed the cattle to walk into the cattle crush, one after another, so I could test each one. This involved measuring the skin thickness on their necks before injecting a small amount of avian and bovine tuberculin into that skin in two spots, one above the other. I would then return three days later to check for swellings at the injection sites. The size of the bovine swelling compared with the avian one would determine whether an animal was that dreaded thing – a 'reactor'. It was not a bad job

– simple and straightforward, free of stress and out in the fresh air. The handling system on the brothers' farm looked good – all the yearlings were corralled at one end of the pen, the cattle crush was oiled and, although old, appeared to be very functional. Just like the farmers, I hoped. Despite the heat, it would be a good morning's work, although while testing cattle it is frustratingly difficult to have a proper conversation, such is the relentless regularity of reading out ear tag numbers, taking a note, injecting and opening and closing the cattle crush. Then there was the number-checking and number-recording. The cattle proved to be gentle and calm, which was a bonus. Sometimes cattle do not like being handled, especially around the head and neck, and jump, rush and kick in a belligerent way, which makes the job much more difficult, as well as quite dangerous for the vet and the farmers.

However, gentle, calm cattle can be frustrating and, handled by two elderly farmers, progress was disappointingly slow. It was taking simply ages to persuade each docile animal to wend its way into the crush and the extra time in the sun was causing everyone to wilt.

'Cush, cush. Come on, that's a good boy, cush cush,' was as much coercion as could be mustered. After an hour, my trousers and shirt were soaked through with sweat and sticking unpleasantly to my body. And the heat was taking its toll on the old boys too.

'I'm going to have to have a lie-down,' one of them kept saying. He repeated this so frequently that it became something of a mantra. I really did think that we should stop for a break. At last, we were down to the last handful in the pen. It was just as well, because both brothers had slowed to a crawl. For my part, every bit of my clothing was wringing wet and my feet squelched inside my wellies in a good centimetre of sweat, which had trickled down my legs and into my socks.

As the last bullock of the first batch left the rusty, old crush and wandered off into the field to join his friends, I overheard the conversation between the two Mr Wilkinses.

'You know, I'm going to have to go and have a lie-down. I'm completely jiggered.'

Jiggered, but at least no one had keeled over so far. Half the cattle had been tested, with just one escapee, which was quickly recaptured. We were progressing very, very slowly and the pace of moving cattle through the system got slower as we all got hotter and wetter, drenched in sweat. Mutterings of 'I'm absolutely jiggered' and 'I'm going to have to go and have a lie-down' punctuated the work with increasing frequency, up to the point where I thought I heard the phrase approximately once per animal, although I wasn't keeping count (I too was jiggered and very hot and, if I was honest, I needed to go and have a lie-down too). Thankfully, as always happens, even in times of great adversity, the end came eventually and the task was completed. We all sat down on some grass, under a small rowan tree in an adjacent paddock that offered a modicum of protection from the blazing heat. I checked a couple of numbers and completed a few more bits of paperwork and then we could all relax. It was hard to say which of us was more pleased to have finished.

I arranged a time to return to read off the test. I reassured the two brothers that it would be much easier than it had been today and wouldn't take so long. They didn't seem convinced as they waved me off before heading to the farmhouse for their long-awaited lie-down. I, meanwhile, had an hour's drive back over the beautiful heather moors to occupy my time. All I needed was to find an ice cream somewhere along the way.

Read-off day was a very busy day and I was much later arriving at the farm than I had arranged (even though in summertime farm animal work is supposed to be quieter, with fewer calvings and sick cattle). By the time I headed out across the moors to meet the Wilkins brothers for the second time, the sun was changing colour and the shadows lengthening and I felt bad for having kept the old farmers in suspense for longer than necessary. While the read-off would be easier than the initial testing, it would also be considerably more tense. If I found any reactions on the necks of the cattle, everyone would become anxious. The measurements were crucial, since if the bovine lump was bigger than the lump at the site of the avian injection, it was likely that this animal was a TB reactor. It would be taken away for slaughter and the herd would be put under restrictions, with the certainty of more tests. At least with evening approaching, it would not be so hot for me and my trousers might stay dry. The brothers should be able to manage without needing to go for a lie-down too. And I had the prospect of seeing the sun set over the heather as I drove home. It was hard to call that work – just as long as there were no lumps! Luckily, for all concerned, especially the old, hot farming brothers, there were no lumps anywhere to be seen. The test was clear and everyone could relax.

Later that same week, I had a serendipitous encounter with another elderly farmer, with whom I had worked many years earlier. He was a character who would never have needed a lie-down, even as he got older.

I had seen an elderly gentleman in a trilby hat, carrying trays of bread and buns in the baker's shop over the road from the practice, and immediately thought he looked familiar. It was the trilby hat. But I was sure it couldn't be my old friend – he'd been a farmer, not a baker, and farmers are creatures of huge habit. I could not have imagined him switching from tending his cattle to baking buns, although I knew he'd retired several years ago. I also knew that he was unlikely to be spending his dotage at the bingo hall or cruising the Mediterranean. He was sure to be keeping himself busy.

My suspicions were finally confirmed when the lady who owned the bakery came in with her cat – a Siamese cat – who had lost his voice and his appetite. She also brought her father along with her.

'It *is* you, isn't it, Bert?' I finally blurted out, as the two of them put the cat basket on the consulting room table.

'Aye, it is Julian! Hoe yer doin'? I keep seein' yer from over t'road and I thought I had bitter come and say 'ello,' Bert replied, in his typically exaggerated Yorkshire accent, which was quite distinct and unlike any other I had ever heard.

Abandoning the job in hand, we spent the next ten minutes catching up and recounting past stories and shared experiences. Eventually, I regained some professional composure, stopped nattering and turned my attention to the Siamese cat. Luckily, it was easy to find his problem. After listening with my stethoscope to the rasping noise from his windpipe and sticking a thermometer up his bum to discover he had a high temperature, I could make my diagnosis. He had a bout of tracheitis. As I drew up the appropriate drugs into a syringe, conversation drifted back to old anecdotes.

Bert was one of the best farmers I have worked with. Like the Wilkins brothers, and many others of that generation, he always wore a proper shirt and jacket, but he also always sported a slightly battered trilby hat. He was the manager at a farm that nestled under the tree-covered slopes of the edge of the Hambleton Hills, outside the picturesque village of Cowesby – an apt name if ever there was one! It was a beautiful farm in a beautiful setting and the ancient stone of both the farm buildings and the houses spoke volumes about its history.

The herd to which he tended was based on the traditional Friesian crossed with Hereford cow. In this system, a Hereford bull was used to get black and white dairy cows pregnant so they would lactate generously, after producing sturdy calves. The female offspring then made excellent suckler cows, as they were quiet, had good maternal instincts and also produced copious amounts of milk (as a result of their Friesian genes) so that their calves would thrive and grow quickly. The cows all looked identical – black and white but with distinctive white circular spots around each eye. A bit like the reverse of a giant panda.

Bert taught me a lot about farming and about the illnesses and ailments of cattle. I used to go to the farm as a young vet not long out of vet school. Bert would always listen to my veterinary opinion, even though he had been working with cows since before I was born. At every visit, though, I made sure I gleaned just a little bit of sage advice from this experienced and wise farmer. It might be a trick to predict when a cow was likely to calve, some useful tips on when to intervene when a cow is calving, or the most sensible approach to managing a down cow – one who couldn't stand up after a bad delivery. Bert knew it all and I sensed he also enjoyed sharing the knowledge he had accumulated over many decades.

Equally, Bert's animated enthusiasm when he witnessed something new, something I had managed to do that he hadn't seen before, was infectious. Admittedly, there were very few such occasions, but one of those occasions was a Caesarean section we did together early one Sunday morning. It was spring, so despite the earliness of the hour, it was light and bright. The sunny yellow daffodils, the snow-white blossom on the blackthorn hedges and the new, fresh greenness to the fields made it a joy to be out in a countryside bursting with life.

Bert was certain the calf was too big to be born naturally, and I trusted his judgement. By the time I arrived, he had already prepared a table on which I could place all my surgical equipment, right next to the cattle crush, which would make the job much easier than it often was.

Bert had not seen many operations like this, he told me, because their bull usually produced small, easily delivered calves, which is always a good thing and a sign of well-considered herd management. However, a new bull had recently arrived on the farm and his calves were turning out to be bigger than expected. Bert watched in amazement as I made my incisions through the cow's left flank, through the muscle layers and finally into the uterus, before retrieving the calf's back leg and delivering it into a wonderful springtime world. I remember pulling out the whopping calf and clearing the slime from its nostrils, before setting about the all-important sutures to repair the surgical site as quickly and neatly as possible.

'By gum, that's some fancy work, Julian!' Bert exclaimed, full of praise at my work as he watched me closing the various incisions. 'You can darn me socks if you want, you're that good with a needle!'

As time went on, our mutual respect grew. One morning in late summer, when the suckler calves had grown big enough to be eating a significant amount of grass as well as the final dregs of their mothers' milk, I went with Bert in his tractor to see a calf that was lying in a field, unable to stand. Visiting a patient on a farmer's tractor always added an extra element of drama. I also had to work out in advance what equipment I'd need and which drugs to take with me. It would have been a nuisance to have had to take the precarious ten-minute journey back to my car to retrieve a crucial medication that I had left behind.

The calf was perched at the top of a steep-sided bank, above a little tree-lined beck. Its mother was standing nearby, confused and anxious about her baby and alarmed when a tractor arrived with not one, but two humans, who both peered at her calf.

'I can't make nowt of it,' Bert puzzled, as we both stood, hands on hips, staring at the six-month-old calf. 'I've never seen owt like this before. It was fine this morning. Now it looks like it's abart dead. So that's why you're here! Ti tell me what's up wi' it!'

The appearance of the calf reminded me of a series of unusual cases I'd seen when I worked as a locum in the north of Scotland, right at the start of my veterinary career. Suckler herds were everywhere and I learnt a huge amount about this type of cow in just a short period. I examined the calf carefully. Its temperature was low – a bad but non-specific sign – and its membranes were pale. This suggested anaemia, but the cause was still obscure. Standing in a field, at the top of a bank accessible only by tractor, I knew I'd have to rely on my clinical skills alone, rather than the laboratory tests or ultrasound scans we might employ for a dog or a cat. I listened to the heart, lungs and rumen, palpated the umbilicus and the abdomen as best I could – fluidy and tender – then stuck my finger up its rectum to see what the faeces looked like. The tarry, black and sticky stuff that appeared on my glove gave me the final piece of information I needed to complete the jigsaw.

'Bert, I think this calf has an abomasal ulcer,' I explained. 'It's not very common, but I've seen it before in calves at this age. It's just like when a person gets a stomach ulcer. If it bursts then the outcome is bad. We can try some treatment, but I'm not sure how successful it will be.'

I reached for one of the syringes of medication I'd brought with me.

'Well I never! I've never heard of that in a calf. I'm sure you're right. You'd better try and get it fixed then.' He was as pragmatic and optimistic as ever.

Back in the reality of my consulting room with a sick cat, Bert's daughter was beginning to roll her eyes. Her Siamese cat was still sitting patiently in its basket as Bert continued to recount stories from our past: 'And do you remember – of course y' do – the Kerry cow?'

We both burst out laughing. It shouldn't have been a laughing matter, because the Kerry cow had been down overnight and in a perilous state, suffering from milk fever in a cold and damp field, halfway up a hill. Serious as the problem was, it was straightforward to treat, which was lucky because this was a favourite cow and, more importantly, also a favourite of the boss's wife. The Kerry cow was more of a pet than a member of the commercial herd. The boss's wife had a fearsome reputation. She had a short temper and a sharp tongue and her authoritarian, aristocratic voice was well known by (and struck fear into) many in the farming and equine fraternities of the north. The first time I met her, I had only just started work as a vet and was young and inexperienced. It was one of my first jobs when I arrived in Thirsk and our encounter led to a contretemps that didn't get our relationship off to the best of starts. I had been called to check a litter of newborn spaniel puppies, which was a standard thing to do. It was important to check them for abnormalities and a house visit avoided upsetting the new mum by loading her into the car and travelling to the practice. I listened to each one's heart, checked for cleft palates and confirmed the sex. I felt happy I'd done a good job.

'Now can you do their tails, please?' she asked in a matter-of-fact way.

I must have looked surprised by this request and so she

continued, 'Docking. They need docking. These are working dogs. We always have them docked. We'll never sell them with their tails on!'

This caused me a problem. I have never been a fan of chopping the tails off little puppies. In my opinion, it is an outdated practice and, while there may be a risk of tail injury in an enthusiastic Springer Spaniel when it reaches adulthood, either through excessive wagging due to a general enthusiasm for life or because of injuries from bracken or brambles, I do not see this as justification for cutting off a perfectly healthy part of the body. Dogs can get injuries to their ear flaps, for example, but nobody suggests removing these just in case they succumb to accident later in life!

Anyhow, I was not prepared to undertake the procedure. I explained the situation, my feelings on the matter and the current guidance on professional conduct from the Royal College of Veterinary Surgeons. As you can imagine, this did not go down well. Steam started to emerge from her ears and lightning from her eyes, before her husband stepped in to diffuse the situation. Afterwards, and maybe *because* I stood my ground on that first occasion, we actually became very good friends, and we've since enjoyed many cups of coffee in the farmhouse after a job on the farm or glasses of fizz at social events. But now, let me go back . . .

Back to that foggy autumn morning and the recumbent Irish cow, after the spaniel-puppy-tail incident but still in my early days as a vet. The treatment was simple – a couple of bottles of intravenous calcium were all that was needed; but even after these corrective bottles of medicine had been administered, the cow stubbornly refused to get up.

What is often required in these circumstances is some gentle encouragement. Inertia sets in in the cow, who has often been recumbent overnight, resulting in sluggish reactions and numb legs. The calcium usually provides a very quick solution to the actual cause of the problem. The cow will immediately let out a huge burp as the elixir flows into her jugular vein, which confirms that it is doing its thing, revitalising the muscles and getting the rumen moving again. The Kerry cow burped like a trooper and we both tried to encourage her up onto her feet. Still no response. We really needed her to stand – the longer a cow is down, the worse its chances of recovery. It was dangerous to give more of the calcium solution, so we had to just get physical with the diminutive but obstinate patient.

We positioned ourselves beside the recumbent Kerry cow, uppermost on the hillside, and got ready to gently knee her in the side. Although this does need to be done firmly, it doesn't hurt (well, it does – it hurts the knees of farmer and vet) and often gives the appropriate impetus for the cow to clamber to her feet. It's a bit like giving her a prod in the ribs.

Just as we were ready to go and counting down from three, Bert suddenly whispered, 'Ey up! She's coming!' And with that he immediately stopped what he was doing, urging me to stop too. He tipped his head in the direction of the farm buildings, just as the boss's wife appeared at the gate, marching in typically belligerent fashion towards her cow and us.

'This is her favourite cow,' Bert hissed, under his breath. 'She'll kill us if she sees us doing that! She's sure to think it's cruel and we'll both be in the doghouse! You'll have to offer some gentle words of encouragement rather than knee her in the ribs!'

Bert changed his tack: 'Cush, cush little girl, up you get. That's a good little girl.' He was a wise farmer and not for the first time, nor the last, I was very happy to be guided by Bert's experience and his words of wisdom.

14. Roger, Robert, Richard and David

Farming is often a family affair, a business handed on from generation to generation. A father works alongside his son, daughter or grandson.

Sadly, in these modern times, traditional cross-generational working patterns are not so common. My first experience, and probably one of the best examples of different generations of a family working in unison, was at a fantastic farm just outside Grassington, in the heart of Wharfedale. I had the chance, during my university holidays, to spend a month learning the intricacies of dairy and sheep farming at Hall Farm – a typical Yorkshire farm if ever there was one.

John, the father, worked alongside his two sons, Jonathon and Angus, and the boys' grandfather helped out, too. I was fortunate to benefit from their experience and the short spell I spent there was hugely influential on me in the early stages of my veterinary education.

I loved the jobs I was given – feeding the calves with milk first thing of a morning, bedding up the young stock, scraping out the cubicles and visiting the heifers in outlying grazing with Angus to check if they were bulling. This involved a Land Rover journey to the field, where we would watch the heifers every day for about half an hour. Any cattle showing signs of oestrus would be noted and we'd collect them up into a small pen to allow them to be artificially inseminated. This is a technique to get the young females pregnant to a bull with specific characteristics suitable for first-time mums – for example, a bull that produces small, easy-calving calves.

A small volume of semen would be injected into the heifer's uterus by Angus or his brother and I would watch, enthralled at the making of a new life; a new generation of cattle about to begin. It was hard to call it work, sitting in the sun-drenched passenger seat of the 4x4, or wandering amongst the heifers, and I loved every minute.

I got to grips with the insides of a milking parlour, although the responsibility of milking the cows was too much for a temporary farm-helper like me. I'd help bring the cows in from the fields for milking and help take them out again. One hundred cows walking along the road, trying to eat garden shrubs and flowers, is not a sight we see very often these days. In busy times, when everyone is in a rush, it's hard to imagine this happening at all – impatient car drivers having to travel for half a mile at the pace of a Friesian cow! Yet in Threshfield – a village in Wharfedale – in the September of 1993, this happened four times a day as cows came and went, morning and evening, from the fields where they were grazing to the milking parlour and back.

Between helping with milking and checking the heifers for signs of bulling, the three generations of farmers made use of my extra help to mend some of the drystone walls so characteristic of the area. Somewhere along the road from Pateley Bridge in Nidderdale, up and over the great bulk of Greenhow Hill, through Hebden and to Grassington, the village just before Threshfield, there is an imperceptible change from dark gritstone drystone walls to pale, limestone ones. It was the paler stone that I was using, as I tried my best to match stones from the pile near my feet to the holes in the walls we were trying to mend. It was painstaking work and progress was slow, but we chatted incessantly about everything to do with the farm and farming. I was like a sponge for knowledge, although I didn't really learn how to mend a hole in a drystone wall. I loved being outside, in the fresh air of Yorkshire, and, at least for a few weeks, I was an extended part of this multigenerational family.

My favourite job while working at Hall Farm was gathering the sheep from the moor. September was the time when ewes and lambs would be brought in off the hill. Old ewes had their mouths checked to see if they were fit enough to endure another winter, have another set of lambs and rear them successfully on the wild hills. Wonky or missing teeth, lameness or imperfections in the udder meant it would be too tough for the ewes to have another year on the fells and rearing another crop of lambs would be difficult.

We sorted out and weaned the lambs that had been running with their mothers all summer. The lambs were called 'mules' – cross-bred sheep, the result of mating tough Swaledale ewes with the exceptionally ugly Bluefaced Leicester tup. These utilitarian animals made superb mothers, so the gimmer (female) lambs would be sold to the lowland flocks further south, where they would be mated with 'terminal sires', like Suffolks or Texels, to add muscle to their offspring. I always find the phrase 'terminal sire' an odd one. Usually in the context of my work with animals this would mean a sire with an incurable illness. It means nothing of the sort, in fact. A 'terminal sire' is the basis of the sheep breeding system, fathering lambs which are perfect for the butcher's shop and the Sunday dinner table. The mules bred in this part of Yorkshire would be dipped and then sold at the gimmer lamb sales in Skipton, where sheep farmers from the south would gather to buy new stock to enhance their flock for the forthcoming breeding season. I loved it all, although the dipping process, where the poor youngsters would be submerged in an acrid-smelling chemical bath to kill parasites and stain their fleeces a more appealing colour, was not so nice to be involved with.

So, when I met Roger and his sons, Robert, Richard and David, a farming family who lived in the foothills of the Pennines, memories of my time, twenty-five years earlier, working alongside several generations of tough Yorkshire farmers in Wharfedale came flooding back.

The first time I had met them was in unusual circumstances. Circumstances that involved a film set, about six cameras, extra lights, famous television presenters with autocues and even a green room! It was all part of a television series called *Springtime On The Farm*, produced for Channel 5 by the same production company – Daisybeck Studios – who make *The Yorkshire Vet*.

Springtime On The Farm was filmed over a week and based at Roger and his sons' farm, Cannon Hall Farm. I'd been asked to participate as a 'special guest', although I was not really sure I was entitled to that description. My role was to sit on a straw bale and comment on some of the veterinary aspects of farming, and I was scheduled to do two stints during the week of filming. I had got used to being in front a camera in *The Yorkshire Vet*. However, that only involved a single PD (producer-director) pointing the camera at me, and a single sound assistant with a big, fluffy boom. First Laura, then Ross, had been my near-constant companions over the preceding four years and it no longer really felt like I was on telly. Talking to Laura about what I was doing, while calving a cow, was more like chatting to a friend than being interviewed for a broadcast to over two million people on national television. Sitting on a bale, in front of *proper* TV people like the presenters Adam Henson and Lindsey Chapman, with multiple cameras, some attached to swinging booms, being filmed live, was a very different experience and quite nerve-wracking. It was also quite a lot of fun.

I was introduced to Roger and his sons before we went on air. We chatted for half an hour or so in the green room, during which time I learnt much about their farm. The green room is, rather disappointingly, not green at all. It is simply the room (usually small, but on this occasion large) where the TV 'talent' congregates to go through the format of the show, check timings, confirm the topics to be discussed and so on. It is also a place to drink coffee and wait for a slot in make-up. I would never have imagined that ever in my life I would be waiting for a slot in make-up! Four years ago, my only knowledge of this world was from brief mentions on *The Graham Norton Show* – a favourite programme of mine – where stars would talk about chatting and sharing a glass of wine in the green room. It sounded like a mystical place, full of glamourous Hollywood A-listers. But, by the time I got to *Springtime On The Farm*, I had experienced enough green rooms to know they were unlikely to hold as much glitter and razzmatazz as I had once imagined (although I did once meet Janet Ellis from *Blue Peter*, AND Bucks Fizz, the 1980s pop band, in one). Today I was sharing the green room with some Channel 5 commissioners and producers, J.B. Gill from the boy band JLS and a collection of farmers who were contributing to the show, variously assembled from Yorkshire and further afield. It felt rather surreal.

I watched the VT clips of what was to follow in the show, so I knew what we would be discussing. One of them recounted the history of Cannon Hall Farm. It described how Roger's father had died suddenly while Roger was still at school, and how Roger had worked hard to make the farm pay. But the challenges of making a living through traditional farming had become too much and so he, with his three sons – Robert, Richard and David – had grasped the nettle and worked together to transform the struggling business into what it was now – not just a farm, but also a visitor attraction, offering the public an insight into the actual workings of a modern mixed farm. It was the perfect example of different generations of farmers within a family working together, with a common aim, to make a superbly successful enterprise. It was also the perfect place for *Springtime* (as everyone connected with the series quickly dubbed it) to be based.

I was 'miked' up, with radio transmitter in my back pocket, just like I had been every day of filming for *The Yorkshire Vet*, but I was out of my comfort zone and the adrenalin was beginning to flow. Just as I was about to go onto the straw-bale stage, I sensed a small commotion amongst some of the production team. A walkie-talkie was jabbering away and through the crackling intercom, from where I was standing, I could just make out the nature of the problem – a ewe had lambed up at the lambing shed and had prolapsed her uterus. A prolapsed uterus is a life-threatening condition. David was holding the organ in place, but the ewe desperately needed some veterinary attention and, luckily for her (and for me – at least I would be reacquainting myself with the comfort zone that I had been about to leave), I could provide the treatment she needed.

'I should go and help,' I suggested to the man with the walkie-talkie. 'I have my stuff in the car. I can have it sorted in fifteen minutes. It's a serious problem and I think it's important that I go and sort it out.'

As I headed to the car to retrieve my kit, presenters and producers alike started wringing their hands and making strange faces and noises of objection. 'We're just about to go on air! We can't change the schedule now! The sheep will have to wait. We're on in five!'

I was in a conundrum – I had the skills and the equipment to save this sheep, which was just at the other end of the farm. The lads could call their own vet, but the surgery was a full half an hour away, so it would be at least forty-five minutes before anyone arrived. I knew what I should do, but the TV guys didn't want to upset the apple cart. Or the schedule.

Luckily for the sheep, and for me, a rotund and enthusiastic man came running to the rescue. Paul Stead was the MD of Daisybeck Studios and executive producer of the show. He had heard the news of the emergency and was running as fast as he could, which was quite fast for a round man, with his ID card flapping around his neck and two telephones, one in each hand. I could hear him even from a distance, although one of his phones was being used to contact me.

'Get up there Julian!' he bellowed, barely able to contain his excitement. 'There's an *actual* emergency. It's a sheep and she needs your help. Never mind the schedule! This is what happens with LIVE telly. It's chuffing TV gold! Thank God you're here!' And with that, I headed up to the sheep, with flagrant disregard for the schedule. I felt like a maverick. A maverick in wellies and waterproof trousers, with a syringe for an epidural and about to save a life!

David and Robert had been on hand in the lambing shed,

supervising the action, as all good sheep farmers do. The ewe in question had just lambed. Her lamb was healthy and the birth was fine, but moments after the lamb appeared the uterus followed, turning itself inside out and prolapsing through the vulva. Luckily, David had spotted it immediately, just as it was about to land on the straw, and, like the boy who put his finger in the dam, managed to hold everything in place.

It was a simple job to administer an epidural, numbing the area and relieving the ewe's urge to strain, allowing me to replace the inverted uterus and suture the vulva to keep everything where it should be. The ewe had enjoyed a lucky escape and so had I – from the first part of the show! I cleaned the ewe, cleaned myself up and made my way back to the straw-bale set and my place in front of the cameras.

'Hello, Julian, welcome to *Springtime On The Farm*,' enthused Adam Henson. 'What have you been up to in the lambing shed just now?'

I knew exactly what to say and could talk freely, without any autocue. Suddenly, cameras or not, I was back in my comfort zone.

It had been a funny old day. Another day when vet work and TV collided. It was something I was starting to get used to!

I must have made an impression upon Roger and his sons on that day, because they asked me back to their farm not long afterwards. It was quite a long way from Boroughbridge. Further than our usual catchment area. That said, horse vets from the practice would sometimes travel fifty or more miles to vet a horse for a client prior to purchase, so it wasn't completely unheard of. I explained that we were too far away to attend emergencies out of hours, and also that they needed to ensure their own vet didn't mind me parachuting in on his client every now and then. I had also, unintentionally, acquired a reputation for being an expert in llamas and alpacas. While I love treating these peculiar but endearing characters, I don't think I am an expert. I do, however, have an enthusiasm for them, and enthusiasm goes a long way. It was to take me a long way soon – all the way down the M1 to Cannon Hall to see Audrey the alpaca.

Audrey had a problem with her teeth and, although she was managing to eat and they didn't appear to be causing her any serious discomfort, they were definitely very wrong.

'It's as if there are *too many*,' Robert had explained down the phone. 'And there isn't enough space for them all. They are pointing in all directions and I'm worried. I'm sure, before long, they'll cause her a problem, so I'd like them looking at and I think you're the man for the job!'

'Okay, I'll see what I can do,' I replied, racking my brains to visualise the problem. I couldn't picture what Audrey's mouth might look like, so it was hard to come up with a plan. Then I had a flash of inspiration.

'Could you send me some photos?' I asked. This would be the most useful way to assess what I'd be able to do. Ross, my cameraman at the time, smelled an interesting story for *The Yorkshire Vet*. For him, it ticked a lot of boxes – a very visual problem, a fluffy and appealing patient and a farmer passionate about his animals. The only missing piece of the jigsaw at this stage was a vet who had a plan about what to do. Removing the extraneous teeth would be difficult and would almost certainly require a general anaesthetic, which was usually to be avoided if possible. I wondered whether I could put a brace of some sort around the teeth, to pull them into alignment – I'd done something similar in the past, of course, to stabilise a fractured jaw in Dobbie the llama, but that had been a temporary arrangement to let the fracture heal and I wasn't certain it would work as a permanent solution to wonky teeth. Hopefully the photos would shed light on Audrey's dental issues so I could come up with some sort of plan before I headed south.

'That is a good idea, Julian.' I could hear relief in Robert's voice. 'I'll take some this afternoon and send them over. My dad is at a loose end, so he can help me. It would be great if you can sort something out. The teeth are not causing a big problem now, but I am really worried that they will before too long.'

I waited, over the course of the afternoon, for the ping of my WhatsApp with the all-important pictures. What appeared on my phone was a selection of images of a very odd-looking alpaca. Audrey looked like something between Ken Dodd and Austin Powers, with a mouthful of teeth pointing in all directions. I wasn't sure what I could do, but quickly replied to Robert to say that I was happy to come and help and that I'd do my best, but couldn't promise anything.

'Oh, and by the way. Would it be all right if I bring Ross with his camera?' was my final question.

A week later, and after a few telephone conversations with Cannon Hall Farm's own vet, Matt (who was quite happy for me to chip in and help), I headed south to the farm. When I arrived Ross was already there, capturing endearing shots of the patient and asking Robert and his family about Audrey. Even from the far side of the barn, as I got out of my car, it was clear that Audrey had a mouthful of extra teeth.

'Can we have a closer look?' I called as Robert and Roger strode across to meet me. I needed to keep Audrey still so I could examine her troublesome mouth in more detail.

Audrey was easily coerced into a cattle crush. Although it was not specifically designed for the job, it worked well to restrain her. Not that she needed much restraint. She was clearly used to being handled and, from the very outset, was impeccably behaved. Normally alpacas and llamas do not like their faces or heads being touched, so I had been anxious about how Audrey would react to my examination, but she didn't mind at all.

I peered into her mouth and counted all the teeth. Alpacas, like sheep and cows, only have front teeth on the bottom jaw. The upper jaw has a hard, rubbery pad on to which the lower incisors abut, to allow grass and other herbage to be grasped and nibbled. Audrey had eleven incisors in total. There should have been six. The only plausible explanation was that Audrey had retained five of her baby teeth, which should have been pushed out as the adult teeth emerged, just as they are in humans. Her adult teeth had obviously erupted next to the baby teeth, leaving a mouth bursting with teeth.

'What are you going to do?' asked Ross, prompting me for an explanation to give to the viewers. It was an apt question and not one to which I had an immediate answer.

'I'm not sure, to be honest, Ross,' I replied, not taking his bait for a line for telly.

After a bit of pondering, I came up with a plan. I decided to use special wire – the same wire I would use to saw off a cow's horn – to slice off each extraneous tooth at its base. They were all too solid to remove completely without a full anaesthetic to loosen the roots, and this would be too risky for the alpaca. By wiring them off, I would avoid the need for a general anaesthetic. In fact, I would not need any kind of anaesthetic, because the incisor teeth of camelids do not have any nerves. The process would be completely painless.

Just quarter of an hour later, I had a handful of alpaca teeth and Audrey's mouth looked much more normal.

'That's 50p's worth there in your hand,' commented Robert. Obviously, the tooth fairy of South Yorkshire was much more miserly than her North Yorkshire counterpart – in our house five teeth would have raised £5!

We let Audrey out of the crush and she trotted off to join her mates, with her new smile and improved appearance. As we watched, she grabbed a mouthful of hay and started munching happily, as if nothing had happened. The procedure had gone spectacularly well. I handed over the teeth and waved the boys goodbye, wondering what they would have in store for me next time . . . .

15. 'I'm Absolutely Fine'

I had looked after Sid for all of his life. At first, he was a normal, healthy, happy cat who liked to play and do all the things that cats do when they are young.

He came in to see me one evening when he was about a year old. Christine, his owner, was worried about her favourite cat, but couldn't quite put her finger on the problem. Christine lived near Thirsk, but she worked in Harrogate and didn't finish until after five o'clock, so she always arrived at the very end of evening surgery, just as we were beginning to think we might be able to go home!

'I don't really know what to say, Julian,' she explained. 'He's just *not right*.'

As usual when given this description of a patient, my heart sank slightly. There is a multitude of things that can make a cat 'not right', ranging from mouth pain due to sore gums to a stomach or intestines full of cotton thread, a cat-bite injury, infection in the kidneys, having been hit by a car, laryngitis – the list goes on and on. In most cases, we can start to get an idea from the nature of the signs; a cough would indicate a problem in the lungs or at least part of the airways; diarrhoea obviously points to the bowels, while pain when being handled might suggest some sort of trauma. The history also gives us some huge clues. If a cat has been out all night and is not well the next morning, we suspect an accident sustained during its nocturnal adventures – a brush with a car, a fight with another cat or maybe poisoning from misplaced antifreeze. Sometimes a cat who is 'just not right' has just a minor ailment, but sometimes it is life-threatening in its severity. When the cause is not immediately apparent we could be dealing with either option. And cats have an uncanny (and rather annoying) knack of hiding their symptoms, making it harder for a vet. They like to pretend they are normal.

A cat hiding its symptoms reminds me of an incident I had at a family party when I was about sixteen. It was Christmas and my gran and I had enjoyed one too many glasses of Irish whiskey after dinner. I had an especially fond relationship with Gran, who lived just ten houses up the street from my parents' house in Castleford. My grandfather had died a few years earlier, when I was about eleven, and I'd taken to spending quite a lot of time with her. I'd listen, entranced, to her stories of how she'd earned an MBE and visited the Queen, and I loved learning her ways with animals, especially dogs. We were good friends and shared an optimistic outlook on life, taking each day by the horns and getting the most out of every minute. On this particular day we had, between us, extracted most of the whiskey out of a bottle of expensive Bushmills. It was Christmas, after all. By the end of the afternoon we were both pretty plastered, but stalwartly defied any accusations.

'I'm absolutely *fine*, Mother,' I repeated, again and again, when asked if I was okay.

'Catherine, he's absolutely *fine*,' Gran would confirm to my mum, in a carefully controlled reassurance.

It was clear to all concerned, especially after I'd been sick in the pond (or was it the children's sandpit?), that neither of us was fine at all. We spent the rest of the evening asleep in the car to avoid upsetting the other party guests.

So, when I'm faced with a cat, clearly poorly, but stubbornly sitting in the middle of my consulting room table with its normal temperature and no clues suggesting the cause of the problem, I often imagine it stubbornly and defiantly repeating those words that Gran and I used to defend ourselves all those years ago: 'Julian, I'm absolutely *fine*.'

On this day, Sid emerged slowly from his basket and sat, stock-still, on the table. 'Julian, I'm absolutely fine,' he would have said if he could have talked. But, of course, he couldn't, and so I set about trying to work out what was the matter with him.

'He doesn't want to move,' reported Christine. 'He just sits around all day. He eats a bit, goes to the toilet but something's not right.'

I didn't know it then, but (to misquote a line from a book I used to read to my kids when they were small) the words '*Something's not right with Sid*' would be a regular refrain over the next seventeen years of my veterinary career.

The first part of my examination led me directly to the problem. Sid's gums and the membranes in his eyes were horribly pale. He was anaemic and this accounted for his lethargy and inertia. He most definitely was not fine. I showed his pallid gums to Christine, who recoiled in horror – his membranes were so pale they almost looked translucent. I took a tiny blood sample, to allow me to investigate the reason for this while not depriving him of too much of his precious blood. The way he looked suggested he needed every drop and every red cell he still had, and I didn't want to steal any more than the bare minimum.

When I was still at vet school, I spent a summer in America, studying at the University of Pennsylvania Veterinary Hospital. It was an excellent place to learn and I took every opportunity to tap into the huge pool of knowledge that existed there. Everything was done very thoroughly and to a very high standard. Every patient had X-rays, scans, blood tests – you name it and the patients there had it. Such was the zeal for getting a definitive diagnosis that, apparently, some animals underwent so many tests they developed iatrogenic anaemia. Iatrogenic means 'disease induced by the physician'. Iatrogenic anaemia is a shortage of blood brought about by overzealous blood sampling. Ever since then, I have always been acutely aware of this potential problem, especially in complicated cases or in small dogs or cats and when there is already an obvious blood cell shortage.

I explained the situation – Sid was pale and this was highly likely to be due to a shortage of red blood cells. In simple terms, this was either because of blood loss (for example, bleeding externally or internally, or into the bowels), blood cells not being made at a sufficient rate (in the case of bone marrow disease, or iron deficiency), or blood cells being destroyed excessively or prematurely (a disorder called immune mediated haemolytic anaemia, or IMHA). My priority was to work out which of these was going on and what had caused it – and then to embark on some fairly urgent treatment.

When I analysed the sample, the reason for Sid's pallor was clear. His PCV (packed cell volume – a measure of the percentage of red cells in his blood compared to serum and white cells) was just 10 per cent. It should have been four times that. So his blood had just a quarter of the quantity of the vital, oxygen-carrying red cells that it needed. Instead of being a robust red, his blood was like weak orange squash. This was the starting point, but getting to the bottom of the cause might take many more weeks, if not longer.

I started some treatment and arranged for Sid to come in the following day for more tests.

It's fair to say that any cat with anaemia is in a precarious position. Most of the things that cause it are very serious, in particular two viruses called feline immunodeficiency virus (FIV) and feline leukaemia virus (FeLV). If a cat becomes infected with either of these viruses and anaemia develops, then the prognosis is very grave indeed. I prepared Christine for the worst. Explained everything.

Yet, to my surprise, the lab pronounced that Sid was clear of these two nasties. I scratched my head, unsure whether this was an accurate result. Even though Sid was responding well to the steroids I'd given, I wanted to make absolutely certain that there was no FeLV lurking, undetected in his body. The virus can linger in the bone marrow, doing its mischief, evading diagnosis. I arranged to take a bone marrow sample the following week. This time the results were unequivocal – there was no sign of the virus. The tests for IMHA were negative too (I wasn't sure I believed the lab's assertion on this one either). But, Sid's blood count was returning to normal, the steroids working wonders. Although his condition was still serious and I had still not found the cause, we all felt happier. Especially Sid.

As the weeks passed, I checked on Sid every so often. He gradually returned to full health and his blood count came back up to a normal level. Eventually I managed to trim his dose of steroids down to a sensible level. What wasn't trim, though, was his waist. Sid had expanded to become a massive cat, at least partly as a result of the steroids. Viewed from above, he looked like a large egg, his feet hidden underneath rolling folds of fat.

If he sat in a rectangular cat box, his extra tissue flowed to fill every corner so, again when viewed from above, he was actually rectangular. He was enormous, but he was alive and he was very healthy. Very, very healthy but very, very big.

Gingerly, I weaned him off the steroids, carefully monitoring for signs of a falling blood count, but it never came. Sid enjoyed the middle part of his life without medication and his figure gradually returned to normal. However, the weight loss continued, slowly at first but then more significantly. Sid became thin. Then he became *really* thin. His bowels went dicky and his appetite became enormous. It was a classic case of hyperthyroidism, and yet the blood tests showed only marginal elevations in the levels of thyroxine. How and why was this cat defying the normal rules of veterinary medicine for a second time? Much as I enjoyed treating Sid – as much for the cerebral challenge as the satisfaction of achieving a cure – and much as I liked seeing Christine, I was beginning to find the cat's peculiarities mildly irksome.

Sid was the most confusing cat I'd every treated, stubbornly refusing to follow the textbooks and equally stubbornly battling on against all the odds. At the surgery he remained unswervingly aloof, as if deliberately trying to bamboozle me ('I'm absolutely *fine*,' I kept hearing in my head). Even at the very end, he clung on tenaciously. Another rule-breaking illness. As it happened, it was rule-breaking and leg-breaking – it was a fall from the bed. It was rule-breaking because a minor tumble from just a couple of feet onto a carpeted bedroom floor should not result in a fractured femur. And clearly for a weak, eighteen-year-old cat a fall like this was never going to be trivial. There were many tears, from owner and vet, after the final conversation over Sid. He had been a truly amazing cat and one that would stick in my mind for a long time.

Despite Sid's demise, I still saw Christine regularly with her other cat, Milly. Milly had suffered from joint stiffness for most of the second half of her life. She was as stiff as her friend Sid had been fat, but she was a happy cat and her arthritis was fairly well controlled with a concoction of medications, some of which took the form of regular injections. I came to know Milly almost as well as I had known Sid, my diagnostic nemesis. She was, in fact, the second stiffest cat I had ever met in my twenty-odd years of being a vet.

The cat who claimed the title of the stiffest cat ever was one I saw many years ago, and one which should have featured in a veterinary magazine. As its freshly developed X-ray film was hung, dripping, over the illuminated viewing screen, the assembled staff – vets and nurses – gasped in awe and wonder. This was back in the days before digital X-ray processing, when we would have to incarcerate ourselves in a darkroom and fumble around, trying to remember which tanks of noxious chemicals the exposed film needed to be dipped into first, and for how long. The processing time was temperature-dependent, so on a cold day we had wait in the pitch black for what seemed like a lifetime before the celluloid films were ready to remove from the tanks. If we were fastidious, we would check the actual temperature of the chemicals with a thermometer – like the ones used in greenhouses to make sure tomato plants aren't too cold – before we started. If we weren't, we'd estimate how much extra time to leave the films in the fluids, which sometimes worked and sometimes didn't. If the chemicals from one tank got dripped into the next, the films would take on a sepia tinge, just like a family photo from Victorian times. It was also bad if the fixer wasn't used correctly, because then the image would slowly fade, like Marty McFly in the movie *Back to the Future*. There was a lot that could go wrong, which was embarrassing and annoying in equal measure, particularly if we had to send the films off to an expert for an opinion on a confusing chest film or a wonky pelvis.

Anyhow, *the* stiffest cat was from those days – the days of actual X-ray film, the days of movies about futuristic time-travelling cars and the days of poorly balanced diets for cats. This patient had enjoyed a diet comprising exclusively liver. While this is tasty for a cat, it is hopelessly unbalanced and has a very high level of vitamin A. Cats are very sensitive to vitamin A, which builds up in their system and leads to a severe toxicity. One of the effects of this toxicity is the fusion of the bones of the vertebral column, and that is what we saw on the X-ray. The poor cat was completely unable to bend its back, from its head to its tail. It was a sad case, with little hope of a successful cure, but it stuck in my mind as a lesson: DO NOT FEED YOUR CAT A DIET OF ONLY LIVER.

Luckily, Milly's stiffness was not vitamin A related and my regime of treatment meant that she was able to enjoy a happy, relaxed life, mainly on the sofa next to the fire. She was missing Sid, her lifelong companion, but her sedate lifestyle was not badly compromised by being the sole cat in the household.

Some months later, though, I received a text message from Christine, which went like this:

Have you seen the little male cat in your surgery? He reminds me so much of Sid. If nobody claims him, I would love to give him a home. He is Sid's double.

I hadn't actually seen the cat to whom Christine referred, as I had been away in London doing some filming with an animal charity.

'I'll have a look,' I typed as I headed into the kennels to investigate.

Sure enough, there was the cat. It looked about eight months old and had been wandering around a village near Boroughbridge for about a week. Notices had been put up asking if it belonged to anyone, and it had spent a few days in someone's garage having food and attention lavished upon it. Its foster carers, as it were, then arranged to bring it into our practice to check if it had a microchip. But no luck. It wasn't identified by microchip or a collar, so we turned to Facebook. Social media is a brilliant way to disseminate information (be it factually correct or otherwise) and is a superb way of reuniting a lost cat or dog with its owner – or, in this case, finding it a new home. Christine had seen the picture on the practice Facebook page.

'Of course,' I tapped into my phone. 'As long as there aren't any actual owners who come forward. I'll put your name on the kennel.' Then I added, 'he's very cute!'

Over the week, nobody came forward to claim the little stray cat, so we arranged for Christine to come and collect him. It seemed like fate. I hoped stiff Milly would approve of her new friend. I also hoped he would be healthier and less confounding than his predecessor! As it turned out, this little waif was not a problem-free cat either, and his first few months with Christine were punctuated with multiple visits to the vets. But those are stories for another day.

16. Under the Microscope

It was the usual Sunday morning start. Quarter to eight and a sick patient. This time it was a cow with toxic mastitis at one of our dairy farms. I got there as fast as I could, as time was very much of the essence. It was actually my weekend off, but I owed a colleague a Sunday on call, in return for one she had worked for me a few weeks earlier. We all try to help one another by swapping weekends or night duties when necessary, but swaps like this always lead to a somewhat pointless comparison of who has had the busiest weekend. Time would tell how this Sunday swap would go, but so far it was looking like a good deal for Emma.

The cow was very sick and unable to stand. Her head was lolling on the straw bedding of the calving pen and her udder appeared to be changing colour almost in front of my eyes, from a healthy pink to poisonous purple. Acute, toxic mastitis is a serious problem and one that all dairy farmers and cattle vets dread. The arrival of this sudden and aggressive infection in an udder full of milk can, in some circumstances, be fatal. Quite quickly, the toxaemia causes the cow to be very poorly and the farmer to panic. After various intravenous injections and a small prayer to the god of cows (she would need all the help she could get) I headed back to the practice.

My beeper stayed mercifully silent, but there was a cat in the kennels who needed some breakfast. It was the little homeless cat that looked like Sid. He had been with us for a while and no one had come forward to claim him. Christine was delighted. We had neutered him on Friday and he was spending the weekend recovering at the surgery before going to his new home with Christine and stiff Milly on Monday. I also had a mountain of paperwork to plough through; it was getting bigger and bigger as my working days became busier and busier. Easy as it was to put off, Sunday seemed a good time to catch up on the tedious stuff, as there was much less chance of being interrupted or distracted.

But Emmy, my faithful Jack Russell, had other ideas. She'd missed out on her morning walk because of the visit to the cow and she sat expectantly, looking up at me with her impatient but appealing eyes.

I didn't put up much of a fight. 'Oh, come on then. Let's go for a walk,' I said, pushing my insurance forms to one side. Insurance forms are the bane of my life, and I just couldn't face them on a Sunday morning, at a time when all sensible people were still in bed. Emmy jumped excitedly into the car and I drove down to a small car park next to the river. As I pulled in, my path was blocked by a lady standing right in the entrance staring up at a tree, admiring its lovely orange leaves. She was utterly oblivious to my presence. I was tempted to peep my horn, as the back of my car was still sticking out into the road, but I thought better of it – the road was quiet and it seemed a bit rude. Eventually the lady spotted me, raised an apologetic hand

and let me pass. I parked the car and Emmy leapt out with a squeak of excitement. To my surprise, the lady who had just been in my way let out a similar noise and grabbed her husband's arm with one hand.

'It *is* you, isn't it?' she gasped, covering her mouth with her free hand. 'You are the *actual* reason we are here! Derek, I can't believe it! Look who it is! It definitely is you, isn't it?'

I instinctively looked over my shoulder, towards the river behind me. There was nobody else, other than my dog and me, in the car park, so I guessed it must be me causing the excitement.

Shirley (she had quickly introduced herself and her husband) went on to explain, bursting with enthusiasm, how they were visiting North Yorkshire from their home in Essex, how they'd been staying in a hotel in Thirsk and how I was, in fact, genuinely the reason for their visit. Their next stop was to be the practice where I worked. They'd seen me in *The Yorkshire Vet* and were massive fans. No wonder they were so excited to see me. Despite Emmy's impatience, we chatted for quarter of an hour or so and, before I set out on my walk along the river, I pointed them in the direction of the best coffee shops in town and the practice. It seemed to make their day!

Encounters like this have become more and more frequent over recent years. While I suppose I have got more used to it now, being recognisable and being spotted is still very bizarre. The very first time I was asked for a selfie was one Monday while the first series of *The Yorkshire Vet* was on. I was in Thirsk Market Square. 'Ah, my favourite vet,' bellowed a man. 'Can I get a selfie? My daughter is a massive fan of yours and this will make her very jealous.'

The man, Tony, who was a fishmonger from Grimsby – a photo with the fishmonger! I knew I'd hit the big time! – became a good friend. He was always in town on a Monday, which fortunately coincided with both my afternoon off and the day Anne worked late. I'd usually call to see him to buy some of his lovely fish.

It got better (or worse, depending on how you look at it) as time and episodes and books went by. The regularity with which Channel 5 showed the programme didn't help my privacy much. By the end of series seven, we had made nearly a hundred episodes and they seemed to be repeated on an almost endless loop. Every time I visited my parents, Mum would announce: 'Oh, I've just been watching you on telly. It was the one with you and the cow with the so-and-so/sheep with the lump/lovely farmer with the alpacas/swan with the wing/ferret with the alopecia/pig with its overgrown feet . . .' and so on. She developed an encyclopaedic knowledge of each story and each episode, feeling duty-bound to watch whenever I was on – in her words, 'just in case no one else is watching'!

Airports are another place where I really should wear a fake moustache and a pair or dark glasses to retain some privacy. Recently, while passing through Leeds Bradford Airport on the way to a family holiday, I was pulled to one side for a frisk-search. I'm not sure that's the proper name for it, but that was what it was, the security attendant patting his way down each side of my body to my ankles and then back up to my armpits. On his return journey to my armpits, the enthusiastically efficient chap, his face just centimetres from mine, simply said: 'Yep, you're all clear. Good to go. By the way, I love your show.'

On one occasion, I was recognised while travelling down the A19 towards Thirsk. It was during a sad period, when I was contemplating the future. It was late on a spring afternoon. Lambs were skipping in the fields around Leake Church. The eleventh-century church and its neighbouring manor house are all that remain of the medieval village of Leake. They stand in picturesque countryside beneath the escarpment of the moors, just set back from the busy road that joins Teesside and the north-east to Thirsk and places further south. The church is a very beautiful sight for all those commuting up and down the dual carriageway every day.

Anyway, on this day the sun shone low over the fields and the hawthorn hedges looked resplendent in their snowy blossom. I began to recollect past encounters on visits to the farms in the area. There was the cow at Arthur's farm one Sunday afternoon when I was on second call. Ben, the vet on first call, was busy and I'd been sent out as a matter of great urgency. The cow had burst a big artery while she was calving and both she and Arthur were in a pickle. I'd dropped everything and rushed along the tiny lanes, arriving just in time to clamp the vessel with some forceps before the stricken animal bled to death. I remembered the early-morning calvings at Kepwick, struggling with an elderly farmer, in a dimly lit cowshed, straw bedding so deep that we had to stoop to avoid banging our heads. His oversized cows never seemed to be able to get their babies out by themselves and it always seemed to be a night when I was called.

And then there was the cow, stuck and unable to stand, high on a hillside overlooking Boltby. The farmer, Brian, and I had trekked across the moor for about a mile, stumbling over bilberry bushes and heather, to get to the recumbent patient so that I could administer the all-important calcium injection that would give her the impetus to get up and extricate herself from the mire in which she was stuck.

There were other cows, too, including those that had once belonged to my old friend Jeanie, and who, when the time came for her small herd to be sold, had been bought by a nice chap called Ian to join his large herd, which he kept on the edge of the moors. He'd called me one day, not long after the cows had arrived.

'Can you just give them a check over, please?' he asked, slightly apologetically. 'One's got a touch of diarrhoea. I wouldn't normally trouble a vet for something mild like this, but I feel like I've got an extra "duty of care" to these ones. Jeanie thanked me for having them and I promised I'd look after them especially well, so I'd be grateful if you'd give 'em a look over.'

I could just see Ian's farm from the busy road on which I was travelling, and memories of this and other cases came flooding back. By then, as negotiations over the sale of the practice ran on apace, I knew I would not be setting foot on some of these farms again. I could not hold back my emotion and tears flooded down my face. I was crying like a baby as I trundled along in the slow lane. Just at that moment a pickup passed me, full of passengers. It slowed in the busy traffic, allowing me, unknowingly, to catch up. A movement caught my eye – all the passengers were cheering, waving, taking photos and giving me the thumbs-up! I was still tearful – it was hardly the image that was portrayed on telly of the endlessly upbeat, enthusiastic vet. They were seeing me at my lowest, at a time when I thought I was alone.

There seemed to be nowhere I could have any private time or space. Even in my car!

On the whole, the good bits (as always) outweigh the bad, but negative comments from pedantic vets, vet students, veterinary nurses (usually along the lines of 'you shouldn't do it like that!') and people objecting to farming or the pragmatic nature of mixed practice can be very hurtful. There haven't been loads, but it doesn't take loads to cause upset. I once received an email commenting that I had used the wrong type of screwdriver to repair the broken leg of a pug! (The pug, incidentally, made a complete and swift recovery, despite the alleged wrong screwdriver.)

Soon after the first episode of series two, an angry and aggressive email arrived from a veterinary surgeon, a specialist in soft-tissue surgery, working in America. The case that had provoked her email was that of an elderly dog with a huge mass on its side. A colleague had seen this patient as a second opinion from a nearby practice who had taken a 'hands-off' approach, electing not to offer any surgical intervention (or any intervention at all, for that matter). The owners had watched their dog's lump expand to the point where euthanasia was becoming the only realistic option. This was the last thing the owners wanted, but the mass was enormous and probably impossible to remove. In cases like this, the pragmatic vet is faced with a dilemma: to put down a dog that, apart from this huge mass, is otherwise healthy (in which case the dog is *definitely* dead), or to attempt surgery, under general anaesthesia. If it is successful, then hurray, everybody is over the moon; if not, then nobody – neither the owners nor the dog – is any worse off than with euthanasia. The second option also has the advantage that at least it gives a chance of success; owners can feel they've tried everything. If it doesn't work out, the grieving process can be easier.

With this in mind, I try to err on the side of 'giving it a go', provided everyone is happy with this approach. Obviously each case is different, but this time we opted to try to remove the mass. The owners were fully aware of the possible outcome but we all agreed that if we didn't investigate, we would never know. Sadly, the tumour was attached to the area around the kidney and had expanded outwards alarmingly. It was inoperable and, in the face of a seriously challenging anaesthetic and impossible surgery, we euthanised the dog.

Our attempts to do our best for the dog and its owners had been upsetting to the young intern in the US who was studying hard to become a surgeon. I can still remember the words of her irate email:

Under NO circumstances should first opinion vets be attempting retroperitoneal surgery. This is a job for specialists!

It was offensive and unfair. Did she know how experienced I was at retroperitoneal surgery? Did she know that the cost of referral to a specialist was prohibitively expensive for the owners? But it was typical of comments that are, ultimately, upsetting until you get to the point of being able to ignore or disregard them completely. I haven't got to that point yet, even now, some years on.

I spoke recently with Steve Leonard, one of the first 'reality show' TV vets. Steve, who graduated at the same time as I did, was one of the protagonists of the TV series *Vets in Practice*, which followed the fortunes and misfortunes of a cohort of veterinary students through their final year at Bristol Vet School and out into practice. It was a hugely popular series and I had great admiration for the vets involved, for exposing themselves to the viewing public at the very toughest point of their career. Both Steve and I featured on a programme called *Big Week at the Zoo*, and appeared together for part of one of the shows. I felt somewhat out of my depth, as I had very little experience of zoo animals. Steve, on the other hand, as well as being very knowledgeable in the field, was an accomplished presenter in his own right. We chatted over a coffee in the green room afterwards and I asked him about his position as a role model, both for young vets and for people whose previously normal lives had been affected by exposure to the world through television or other media channels. I felt, to an extent, as if I was following in his footsteps – we'd both ended up on television by accident – and that he could probably give me some words of advice.

'How do you find it?' Steve asked, as we discussed the ups and downs of life as a TV vet. 'Being under the microscope all the time, I mean?'

Then he added, 'My lowest point was when a letter appeared in a veterinary journal, from a professional colleague, who slated the programme and everything about all of us. It was a bad moment, but you've just got to develop thick skin and develop it very quickly. Otherwise you would go completely mad! Stick with it, though, if you enjoy it. You bring a lot of happiness to viewers.'

It was a positive endorsement from someone who'd been there before and Steve was completely right. The number of letters, kind messages and excited visitors to both Thirsk and later to Boroughbridge are countless, and show no signs of abating. I met a lady recently in the hardware shop, where I was buying some hooks. There was a commotion by the sink plungers and then the shop owner came over to me, grinning. 'Is it okay if this lady has a photo taken with you?' he asked, 'She's a massive fan and she can't believe she's met you in here. She only came in to buy some firelighters!'

Of course I obliged but, while posing, couldn't help but notice that the poor lady was actually shaking.

'I'm really sorry,' she said apologetically, 'I don't know what's come over me! I'm just really excited.'

She had seemed a very normal lady until the shaking started – life is quite strange these days!

So strange that I found myself at the 2018 National Television Awards, sitting quite close to David Attenborough, Graham Norton and Paul O'Grady. I actually had to walk up the red carpet, which I found a very uncomfortable experience. I've done several live television broadcasts too. The first was on *The Wright Stuff* with the very talented Matthew Wright. I could not have been more nervous, if not terrified. I was completely outside of any comfort zone I had ever had and I didn't like it. However, on the train home to Yorkshire, as is usually the case after overcoming a big challenge, I had a great sense of achievement.

Subsequent appearances have been much less traumatic and the live discussions have not been stressful at all. I've actually started to quite enjoy my periodic trips to London and all that they entail. That said, it's always a relief to get back home and pick up my stethoscope or calving ropes. At least on the farm there are fewer people to cast opinions and fewer reviews of my performance.

Reviews! I'm constantly amused by the reviews. We live in a time where it seems almost impossible to buy anything without having to offer some sort of comment or assessment. In theory this should be helpful – anyone's opinion is valid, surely? Well, you would think so, but a brief look at the reviews that appear on the most-often-used-online-bookseller's website may lead you to question this. Now, I am not obsessed by reading reviews of my own books, nor of social media comments on the TV shows with which I have been involved (Anne begs to differ), but the occasional look – just to catch a snapshot of public opinion – must surely be a useful thing?

'*I bought this for my wife. I think she'll like it. Three stars*' was one comment and review, which I thought was hardly worth making the effort of writing.

'*Five stars. This book arrived on time!*' A good review, but surely more for the delivery service than the content of the book.

'*One star. I did not order this book and I do not want it!*' This suggested a malfunction with the website rather than a bad book, but it ruined my average rating!

'*One star. The words are too small.*'

There are plenty of useful and valid comments there too, but quite a few like this. You have to see the funny side.

Perhaps the most public arena for reviewing television is Channel 4's popular programme *Gogglebox*, where ordinary people are filmed in their homes, watching telly. The point is to see the reactions of these 'ordinary' people as they watch interesting or surprising things from programmes that have been aired the previous week. Ever since the inception of *The Yorkshire Vet*, it had been an ambition of mine to feature on this. It's not often that I get to see people's reaction to what we have made, let alone see it on national television.

The first time *The Yorkshire Vet* appeared on the show came out of the blue. I had got home late on the Friday evening and happened to be perusing the TV listings, checking to see if another programme was on, to work out when to make tea. To my surprise, I saw *The Yorkshire Vet* was listed as featuring in that evening's edition. I got on the phone, hurriedly sending messages to all my producer friends and my family to make sure they were watching. The story featured one of the most dramatic pieces of surgery I've ever done. It was a bull with an enormously swollen eye. The farmer was worried that the eyeball was going to rupture (he was correct) and that it was painful (he was correct on that, too), so I'd taken all the things I needed to attempt to remove it (plus my camera crew). This is quite a challenging procedure on even a cat or dog, under full anaesthetic and in the sterility of the operating theatre, but on the farm, standing in a cattle crush, it was as dramatic and as tense as you would imagine.

I watched the *Gogglebox*ers and their horror as the enormity of the task became clear.

'He's going to have to take it out, Mary,' explained Giles to his wife, in his classic deadpan tone, while the screams and gasps of horror from the other contributors made for great telly.

Watching *Gogglebox* is always funny. Especially watching on the first occasion I featured. We'd been trying to get a spot on this popular programme ever since we started making *The Yorkshire Vet*. The first time we were on was both amazing and exciting. It was implausible to think that our TV series – still a novelty for me – was featuring on another TV programme, with people on TV watching me do my normal job!

We've been on the show several times now, usually with me focusing on the enormous penis of a bull, or the testicles of a donkey, or something particularly gruesome like a huge, custard-filled abscess on a bull! It's started to feel quite ordinary; one evening while Archie, my youngest son, was eating his post-swim-training bowl of porridge in front of *Gogglebox*, he calmly asked between mouthfuls, 'Are you on tonight?', as if it was the most normal thing in the world.

On another occasion, Jack, my eldest, sent a WhatsApp message from the rowing camp he was on, which just said, 'Dad, you're on *Gogglebox*.' I turned on just in time to see that the clip they had chosen was of me collecting a semen sample from a bull. 'I'm so sorry,' I messaged back, 'please tell me you are not with all your friends.' My phone pinged again, and there was a photo of a bunch of teenage boys crying with laughter in front of a hotel TV. It took being an embarrassing parent to a whole new level.

And in one episode of *Celebrity Gogglebox* that I watched, none other than Abbey Clancy commented: 'Oooh, I love *The Yorkshire Vet!*'

Who'd have thought it?

17. It's Not Always Good

The oozing split on my index finger was only part of the reason why the afternoon's visit was distressing, if not downright depressing. The black nail was no longer painful, but the split on the apex of my swollen digit was – very painful. Both had been there for a week. The cause of the persistent throbbing and the intermittent acute stabbing pain had been a llama with a problem chewing its food.

I knew it was stupid to put my fingers in between the llama's molars, but I had needed to ascertain if there was a loose or fractured tooth or an abscess. Maybe there was some sort of growth in there? Whatever it was, it was causing grass and hay to spill out of the right side of the camelid's mouth. In horses or cattle, we have special kit to help with the job of examining the teeth and mouth. Using this equipment, the jaws can be kept open safely for a full and thorough examination. And cats and dogs are usually anaesthetised for dental work; but llamas are an altogether more difficult proposition. I'd managed quite well at the start and concluded that one tooth had now fallen out, but my final check, just to ensure there were no other loose or damaged teeth, was one check too many. The teeth were sharp and serrated and the muscles of the jaw were powerful. The result was a searing pain through the end of my finger. I tried to play down the incident with a muted 'Ouch', but I knew this pain would be with me for a while. As I finished my examination and discussed my findings with the owner of the llama, the latex glove on my hand gradually filled up with blood, like some kind of water balloon, only more sinister.

I made my excuses to visit the toilet and peeled off the glove to inspect the injury. It looked horrible. The nail was already turning purple and there was a nasty laceration surrounded by crushed flesh, right on the tip of my finger. My most important finger, too. I knew that, with lambing time upon us, an injury like this could linger for weeks. Although I could apply skin glue and a hefty plaster, the rigours of veterinary practice at this point in the winter did not lend themselves to problem-free healing. No way.

I searched for something in my car boot to cover up the wound; there was a roll of thin tape somewhere amongst the bottles of medicines and syringes. My fingers were cold and damp and I couldn't find the end of the micropore tape. The thick Elastoplast I usually used for bandaging cows' feet would have to do instead. It made a terrible plaster, massive and cumbersome, rendering my right hand useless for pretty much anything other than holding the steering wheel on the drive back to the practice. Even though the dressing was thick, blood oozed through it. By the time I got back, it was mainly red rather than its original off-white. In theatre, I cleaned the mangled tissue up as best I could and stuck the edges together with some skin glue, which helped, but I knew I was in for a difficult, very tricky few weeks.

So, a week later, I arrived on the farm for what should have been a lovely job. The sun was shining and – although it was so cold that everything metallic was icy to the touch and sucked all warmth from my hands – checking a young bull and pregnancy-testing ten cows was the stuff that young vet students dream of doing. My morning had been busy. An over-full list of appointments had left me short of time, lunch and coffee – the biggest issue. I had another farm visit to do after this one, twenty minutes' drive away, with more cows to pregnancy-test, but I'd reckoned I could squeeze this one in first. It was eminently feasible even in the short days of midwinter, providing everything went to plan. Or so I thought.

But nothing went to plan. I got a sense of foreboding almost as soon as I arrived. There was no farmer to be seen and no cattle ready. I wondered if I'd got the wrong day. I put my wellies on and started to explore the various farm buildings, peering in through doorways and shouting 'hello'. It seemed I was talking only to myself and to the miscellaneous cattle in the miscellaneous sheds.

Eventually the farmer, Geoffrey, appeared from the farmhouse, pulling on his woolly hat. He didn't look very animated and I began to suspect that the job, which should have taken twenty minutes, would be keeping me on the ramshackle farm for much longer. I was certainly going to be late for my next visit and I could feel myself starting to get annoyed as the farmer ambled towards me.

'I've got one to see with pneumonia in a shed over there, but first can you look at this?' Geoffrey said, heading over to a pen of young bulls. He pointed at a rather sad-looking character who was attempting to munch on some hay, but heaving as if he'd just run a marathon. The poor animal's sides were moving in and out like a set of bellows.

'Do you think we should castrate this bull?' the farmer asked, rather to my surprise. I'd been expecting him to ask me for some treatment for the poor thing. If this wasn't the one he thought had pneumonia, I was starting to dread what the one he did think had it might look like. 'I'm going to move some today, to another farm, but if this one goes with them I think I should castrate him first.'

'I don't think that's a very good idea,' I ventured. 'Look at his sides going in and out – he's got chronic pneumonia and I don't think it would do him any good at all on a freezing day like this. If you've got another one with bad pneumonia to look at, it's obviously going around the herd. I think it would be an added and unnecessary stress. I would leave him alone for now, maybe do him in springtime, when he's grown a bit, recovered and the weather's better.' I was trying to steer a sensible course.

'You think it might finish him off if we do him today?' Geoffrey nodded, quite unperturbed. 'Okay, maybe best to leave him 'til another day. Can you have a look at this one now? It's a young calf I've just bought. *He's* had pneumonia too and he's not very well. I've given him some jabs but he hasn't really rallied like I'd hoped. He's over here.' Geoffrey lolloped off to the next building.

The farmer was an ex-city worker, new to farming, and was clearly having some difficulty grappling with the challenges of looking after the herd he had recently taken over. I followed him into the grain store, which was, somewhat unusually, doubling up as a calf shed. Being designed for storing grain, it was obviously less than ideal for housing young cattle. I am constantly surprised at the frequency with which some farmers use buildings to house stock that are completely inappropriate – either unventilated, or dark, damp and draughty – and this was a classic example. I climbed over the piles of wheat, following the rather inept farmer in a two-steps-forward-one-step-back kind of way (which set the tone for the whole visit). It was like walking up a large sand dune. I could see my patient from a distance, lying stiffly on the straw at the back of the pen. His glazed eyes, the abnormal contortion of his body and his bloated abdomen told me we were too late.

'This is him. I think you'll need something strong. Well, stronger than what I gave him, anyway,' explained Geoffrey as he climbed over the gate to try to rouse the calf.

'Oh no. I think he's gone,' he said, surprised and slightly embarrassed, as he prodded the carcass. 'No, it's too late. He's definitely dead,' he confirmed, as the stiff ex-calf stubbornly refused to rise, move or breathe.

We discussed the limitations of the building, the improvements to be made and strategies to counteract pneumonia, our discussions going round and round and on and on until I managed to change the subject: 'I think we should crack on – I have another big visit to do next and I'm already late. Let's get on with the PDs.' Then the crucial question, to which I feared I already knew the answer: 'Is everything set up and ready to go?' I'd seen the all-important cattle crush languishing, inert and inactive in a murky corner of the farm while I was searching for the farmer soon after I'd arrived – which already seemed like ages ago.

'Yes, good idea,' agreed Geoffrey. 'I'll just get the crush organised. There's one cow in that pen, a couple in that pen and eight in that pen.'

My heart sank. Moving the crush, arranging the gates and catching the cattle was sure to take over an hour. And then there was the coercion of each animal into the crush, the palpation of each uterus, the writing down the all-important results on an ephemeral piece of cardboard, torn from the back of a cereal packet, and the outcome and the discussion over what to do with each patient if it was not pregnant as planned. It would be dark by the time I had finished.

I like to help farmers move cattle, operate the crush and so on, but I draw the line at manhandling heavy metal gates to build a handling system from scratch. I like farm work, but what I really enjoy is efficient work; I hate working slowly and wasting time and I hate being late, especially when it is due to someone else's disorganisation. The farmer next on my rounds would be looking at *his* watch in frustration, just as I was looking at mine. I could feel my cortisol elevating to an unhealthy level.

I sat at the open boot of my car, answering emails on my phone as I waited for Geoffrey and a helper, who had just appeared, to organise themselves. Twenty minutes later, the cattle crush had been set up and I put down my phone and pulled on my shoulder-length glove, ready for animal action.

But the farce got worse. Instead of bringing the cattle to the crush, we had to take the crush to the cattle. I tested two heifers for pregnancy in one yard, then stood back in disbelief as all the equipment was dismantled to move to another yard. There was more lugging of cold, metal gates and more tractor manoeuvrings before we were ready to go with the next set of cows. The first was supposedly about to calve. 'Look, she's bagging up,' said Geoffrey, pointing to her udder. 'Do we even need to test her?' I felt inside the cow's rectum. Her uterus was small, fitting into the palm of my hand. She was clearly not pregnant. She was just fat.

'But what about her bag? She's bagging up,' protested the novice farmer, his anxiety rising because, I think, he sensed I was really quite cross with his inept and inefficient system.

'Well, I can assure you, this cow is not pregnant,' I replied curtly, then added, 'Not unless she's been with the bull in the last four weeks.' If the cow had been mated recently, it was possible she might be in the early stages of pregnancy but too early to detect. Good farmers have cows tested five weeks after they've left the bull, so the results of a vet's visit are definitive – pregnant or not pregnant. If the bull is left running with the herd, it's not a very useful test; I'd need to come back again once the cows had been separated from the bull, making this whole afternoon's escapades a relative waste of time.

After much shouting, waving of arms and unsuccessful attempts to corral her, the second cow was eventually caught, but she had managed to shuffle into the crush backward: her backside was where her head should have been and her head at the back of the crush. I'd never seen this before and, although I was cross at the waste of my time, anxious about getting to my next job on time and distracted by the pain in my right index finger every time I used my hand, I found myself chuckling at the ridiculous situation. At least this offered some relief to my ever-rising level of stress. But turning the cow round meant letting her out of the handling system and starting over again. The relief was short-lived as she careered round the pen, determined not to be detained for a second time.

'You know,' I blurted out, 'I think I'm going to have to come back another day when your system is more organised. I should have been at another farm over an hour ago! This is a terrible set-up and, to be honest, I haven't got time to waste like this!'

I knew I sounded rude, but my outburst was triggered by the shambolic lack of organisation and total disrespect for my time. My finger was throbbing, I'd spent an hour and a half on a job that should have taken twenty minutes and I'd only generated about thirty pounds of revenue for my practice.

I considered the ups and downs of my job and of the positives and negatives of working in veterinary practice. Clients' expectations are higher than ever before. Litigation is becoming more frequent, an ever-present spectre lurking in the shadows – in fact, one of the emails I was answering while waiting for Geoffrey to build his handling system was from our indemnity insurer regarding a case brought by a dissatisfied client.

Client complaints are always stressful and, without exception, will ruin a vet's life for a protracted period. It is doubly upsetting when your utmost professional efforts have not been interpreted as such. You have tried your best, done what you believed to be right and yet the client is critical to the point of referring you to your professional body.

How about the little terrier whose nails had been trimmed (at no extra cost) while he was asleep under anaesthetic to have his teeth cleaned, to save the trauma of clipping them while he was conscious? This act of pragmatic kindness backfired for one of my former colleagues. We had not obtained specific permission to trim the nails and the owner went mad when he realised what had happened. His vitriolic reaction involved reporting those concerned to the Royal College of Veterinary Surgeons and informing the local papers, which were only too happy to gobble up a headline-grabbing story. What followed was a horribly traumatic few months for the young vet and nurse. They had just been trying to do a helpful thing.

At least I am a veterinary surgeon with years of practice under my belt and can handle this better than some of my younger colleagues. For a recently qualified veterinary surgeon, such incidents can bring a sensitive soul, desperate to do their best for the animals under their care, to the edge of despair. Many young vets are finding it difficult these days. They often find themselves living alone without the support of a cohort of friends nearby, working too hard, too many days and too many nights, with the omnipresent beeper and unpredictability that comes with being on call. Even for me, the uncertainty of a night on duty – and the lack of control that it brings – is still the hardest aspect of my job. And that is after more than twenty years of being a veterinary surgeon. So much of what we do is out of our control, at the mercy of the beeper, the phone or the whim of the farmer, the disease status of the farm (or even the suitability of the handling system). It's not just the unpredictability, either. The requirement for immediate care can be overwhelming. I heard a story recently from a vet called Laura, who had given up struggling with the pressure. She recounted the story of how, late one evening as she was finishing off a long and demanding round of calls, her mobile rang. She was at the end of a run of two weeks without a night off.

'I have a horse call for you,' explained the practice receptionist over the phone. 'They need you now!' It was the final straw.

'That was the point when I knew I had to stop,' she told me. 'I couldn't continue as a vet, enduring the unrelenting stress and expectation.'

Laura became another statistic; another competent young vet who left clinical practice too early in her career as a result of overwhelming pressure and too many nights on call. And it's always the same. The farmer, struggling to calve his heifer at six o'clock on Saturday evening, needs you *now*. The cat owner, anxious that her cat with chronic, long-standing renal failure has stopped eating, also needs you *now*. At 10 a.m. on Sunday the dog breeder, whose bitch had five puppies during the night, needs a post-whelping check. She needs it *right now*. We care deeply about all these cases, and the more conscientious you are, the greater the load. It rarely seems to ease up.

Busy days packed with challenges are often amazing. They make it a stimulating and rewarding job; we ride on the crest of a wave, curing case after case and helping to bring endless new life into the world. Dynamic individuals thrive on the never-ending stream of sick patients. But sometimes there are too many sick patients, too many interrupted nights. There is insufficient time off, too little time with family or friends. Eventually it becomes exhausting, even for a dynamic type.

I met up with a former colleague not so long ago. She was one of the best vets with whom I've ever worked – dedicated, caring and compassionate all in one. She was a skilful surgeon, a knowledgeable clinician and a lovely person. But she'd been overworked. As staff had left the practice and not been replaced, and as the older partners enjoyed longer holidays, more and more responsibility was placed on her shoulders. She had left the job exhausted, fed up and disillusioned with veterinary practice. On this evening though, three months after she had thrown in the towel, she was happier and more relaxed than I had ever seen her. We enjoyed pizzas cooked in the outdoor pizza oven she and her partner had just finished building, and shared a few glasses of red wine. She smiled all evening.

The volume of work and long hours are not the only causes of disillusionment with the profession. Vets are generally high achievers – we have to get the best results at school and our university course is one of the hardest on which to get a place. Yet much of our work is mundane, and far removed from what we learnt at vet school. While I was trying to persuade a bad-tempered cow into a crush, trying not to stumble over the semi-frozen mounds of straw and cow excrement and trying to ignore my painfully throbbing finger, I considered the university friends of mine who might be sitting in a high-powered business meeting, or operating on the brains of human beings. There are ups, for sure, but there are plenty of downs. Young vets, struggling with student debt accumulated over five or six years, receive, if I'm honest, a shockingly small salary given their level of qualification, training and skill and the number and unsociability of their hours. Is it any wonder that the average length of a vet's career is just seven years, before they jack it in altogether and find another one? And is it surprising that the veterinary profession has one of the highest rates of mental illness, depression and suicide? It is not just because vets have easy access to the strong barbiturates, 'blue juice' as we call it (the blue colour is to avoid confusion with other medications), used to euthanise animals that are suffering. Maybe we have a lighter view of death because we experience it on a daily basis? I'm not sure. One thing is true – all vets have known someone who has done it, or tried to do it, to themselves, just as they have to a dog with terminal mammary cancer or a cat with unmanageable renal failure.

In the past, bouts of depression were blamed on brucellosis. This is a disease of cattle, which causes affected animals to spontaneously abort their calves. We used to have to blood-test cows for brucellosis every two years, usually alongside their TB test. Miraculously, the disease disappeared soon after the foot-and-mouth disease outbreak of 2001. Some suggested it was a lack of DEFRA funds for the testing that coincided with the sudden and unexpected announcement that the disease had been eradicated. However, in the 1950s and 60s, many vets succumbed to the zoonotic effects of brucellosis, or undulant fever as it was called. (Zoonotic is the term given to describe a disease of animal which can be transmitted to humans. They are either frightening or fascinating or both, depending on your perspective. BSE, brucellosis, salmonellosis are just three examples.) Cyclical bouts of night-sweating and depression were the main symptoms affecting those who had contracted the disease from their bovine patients. Was it really to blame for the repeated bouts of mental health problems for vets in this era, or, in the days before it was acceptable to talk openly about mental health issues, was it a convenient excuse? Certainly, despite the eradication of the disease, the incidence of mental health problems has not seen a corresponding decline; our generation of vets cannot blame a cattle-induced bacterial disease for the low points in their week.

Back on Geoffrey's farm, I was annoyed about the futility of my wasted afternoon and anxious about upsetting my next client, but I wasn't quite at that stage. I hoped a deep breath would be sufficient.

Eventually, after various escapees, backwards cows, a couple who refused to be captured, two cows tested twice – the numbers having been transcribed incorrectly on the back of the cereal packet – I was done.

I searched for the bucket of warm water, soap and towel that once would have been provided without a second thought by all farmers, to clean my hands and wellies, but there was none to be seen. I was not surprised when I was waved in the direction of the tap, which ran slowly with icy cold water. Washing my hands under the cold tap was the nadir of a depressing afternoon. But at least the worst part of it was over. At least it had been sunny and at least nobody was injured. Yes, my finger was still throbbing with a constant sharp, stabbing pain, made worse by the chapping effect of the cold water, but that was a mere flesh wound. I clambered into my car and Emmy, my faithful Jack Russell, jumped onto my knee and licked my nose. I was grateful for her unswerving love and loyalty, my constant companion. Late, frustrated, cold and sore, I headed off to do my next job, aiming towards the White Horse of Kilburn, which shone orange in the reflected light of a low-hanging winter sun.

This next visit was to see an old friend. He was organised and efficient and there would be a plan and a system. I rocked up as dusk was approaching.

'Sorry I'm late, Chris,' I apologised. 'I had a bit of a problem at my last farm.'

'Ah, no worries,' he replied cheerfully. 'We're all sorted here. I thought I'd run the bull through first, ring him, bolus him, then PD the cows. I'm all set. I just hope they're all pregnant.'

What followed was half an hour of fun, efficient farm practice. No dramas, no stress – and even the throbbing of my split finger disappeared for a while. Oh, and every cow was pregnant, so Chris was delighted and his excitement rose with each positive result.

Maybe being a farm vet wasn't so bad after all?

And to all the vets out there reading this chapter, gloomy after a lonely day of stressful, hard, underpaid work, with or without a throbbing finger; or to the budding vets-to-be (now worried about their chosen profession) – yes, it can be hard, yes, there are ups and downs, but stick through the downs, because the ups *always* come along. You never have to wait too long. We are lucky to be doing what we do. It's not always good, but (usually) there's more good than bad. It could be worse. We could be sitting, bored, in a board meeting. Admittedly, warm and dry, without cold, chapped hands and a throbbing finger!

18. Quercus and the Party Poppers

Everything was ready for Jonathon's birthday party. Or at least it had been until Quercus, the big, friendly, very unruly wire-haired Pointer intervened with his insatiable and indiscriminate appetite. He had eaten most of the ingredients for the party – sausage rolls, jelly, some of the balloons and, most significantly (for the dog, the vet and the partygoers), all of the party poppers. He had guzzled it all down before anyone could stop him. He had also eaten some cufflinks.

As I cast my eyes down the list on screen of appointments for the afternoon, 'Quercus: eaten party poppers' stood out from the rest.

Vets, nurses and receptionists all gathered to stare at the screen, not knowing what to expect when Quercus arrived and not knowing whether to laugh, cry or panic.

In over twenty years of being a veterinary surgeon, I had never seen a dog who had swallowed one party popper, let alone several.

It sounded like a joke – 'Did you hear the one about the

dog who ate the party poppers? Streamers came out of his bum every time he broke wind!' – but it wasn't a joke and I was worried.

Eventually, the culprit appeared with Jonathon and his mum, Sandra.

'Honestly, this dog!' Sandra exclaimed. 'Everything was going so well and then Quercus got into the kitchen and the next thing we knew, he'd eaten all these things! Is it going to be serious, do you think? Will you need to operate?'

I looked down at the dog with his large ears and slightly droopy eyes and his happy but rather dozy expression. It was hard not to laugh at the situation.

'Well,' I replied, as I started to examine the hapless hound, 'I'm sure we can sort him out, although I've never seen a dog eat party poppers before.' And then, as an afterthought, 'Has he *definitely* eaten them?'

'Yes, I'm sure he has,' confirmed Sandra. 'There was a box of about ten. The box is all chewed up and I can only find three. So, I suppose he might have eaten *seven*! That sounds an awful lot.'

Jonathon had been standing quietly all this time, but at this he piped up, 'Do you think his stomach will explode, doctor?'

'I suppose it might,' I said, mischievously. 'I'd better be careful when I examine him.'

I knelt on the floor, as I usually do to examine large dogs who are too big to lift onto the table. I needed to check Quercus over, starting at his head and working back. First, I looked at his gums, as an obstruction in the intestines would make his membranes change from a healthy pink to a nasty reddish purple. I also wanted to see if there was any plastic or stringy bits of confetti still in his mouth, which might suggest that Quercus had chewed the poppers into pieces rather than swallowing them whole. Either could present a problem. Plastic chewed up into little bits would not cause an obstruction, but the sharp edges could do some serious damage to the wall of the intestine. On the other hand, a whole party popper would simply act as a plug that nothing could get past.

Being a vet is sometimes like being a detective. Of course, animals cannot tell us what is wrong, where it hurts or how they feel – or, as in this case, whether they have *actually* eaten the party poppers. A doctor would simply say to his patient, 'Have you eaten the party poppers?' and the patient would answer, 'No, of course not. That would be a stupid thing to do.' Or, 'Yes, I've eaten seven of them. Is that going to be a problem, do you think, doctor? I'm not sure why I ate them. I just fancied them.' And then the doctor would know exactly what to do.

It's just the same when I see a cat with a limp. If the tomcat could talk, I would ask him, 'Have you been bitten by another cat?' or 'Have you been hit by a car?' and the cat would say 'Yes, that nasty ginger cat from down the road has bitten me on the bottom and it hurts just here . . .' (it would be even easier if the tomcat could also point to the sore bit) or, 'The car just came from nowhere and I couldn't get out of the way in time. I was dazed and confused, seeing stars in front of my eyes. Then I sat in a bush for a while until I felt better and then I came home.' But since animals can't talk, working out where the problem lies is often more difficult, and we have to look for clues. So this was what I was doing with Quercus.

After I had looked in his mouth. I moved to his abdomen, gently pressing with my fingers to try to feel if there were any party-popper-shaped objects in his insides. I needed to be very careful. I didn't want him to explode.

At one time, I looked after all the police dogs for North Yorkshire Police. Some of the dogs were sniffer dogs, trained to sniff out either money, drugs or explosives. When they smelt the stuff that they were trained to sniff, they wagged their tails as fast as they could and stared at the spot where the contraband was hidden. This meant their tails were often sore, so I would see them fairly frequently. The police called the spaniels who sniffed out explosives 'explosive dogs', which always made me laugh. I thought about this as I gingerly examined Quercus's abdomen.

It all felt remarkably normal; I couldn't feel anything hard or unusual. My detective work had, so far, not led me to an answer.

I stood up from the floor of the consulting room, 'I think we will need to do an X-ray,' I explained. The X-ray would show if there were any intact party poppers inside his stomach or bowels. If there were, I would definitely need to operate to take them out, to prevent them from getting stuck. It was possible they could get stuck in either his stomach, his intestines or his anus. There was something else worrying me too. If there were party poppers inside Quercus's stomach, I didn't know how the gunpowder (or whatever the explosive substance was) that made the 'pop' would react with the acid in there. This part of my school chemistry knowledge had left my brain, if indeed it was ever in there in the first place. I tried to recall the exact ingredients of the gunpowder I had made, thirty-odd years ago, in my parents' greenhouse, which did explode when I put a hot metal spatula into it. If only I'd poured some strong hydrochloric acid in, I would have known the answer to the question that preyed on my mind now as I pondered what to do with Quercus. I hoped the same would not happen when it came into contact with his stomach acid.

I also recalled the awful accident that had happened to Mr Secker, the vet in Boroughbridge, in 1902. The packet (or what remained of the packet after Quercus had chewed it) that Sandra had brought in said, of course, that the party poppers should not be eaten, but it didn't say why, or what might happen if you (or your dog) did eat them.

Sandra and Jonathon went home to try to clear up what was left of Jonathon's party, blow up balloons and get more party accoutrements to start again, while I took Quercus through into the kennels to get him ready for his X-ray. He didn't have a care in the world as he trotted behind me, nose in the air, looking for more interesting things to swallow.

He was well behaved for the injection that would send him to sleep, and it was not long before he was sedated, snoozing happily, oblivious to the fuss and worry around him. We lifted him onto the table, arranged him into position and took the X-ray. Within a few minutes, the image started to appear on the computer screen. Several vets and nurses gathered alongside me to peer at the picture.

An X-ray image, or radiograph, is black and white, and various shades of grey. The picture is formed by X-rays hitting a special film, which is similar to an old-fashioned camera film. When the beams hit the film, they make it go black. A film that has not been exposed to X-rays is white. Metal and stones show up very clearly on a radiograph. They appear bright white because the beams cannot penetrate them, and therefore don't reach the film. Air also shows up very well, for the opposite reason – because X-rays travel through it very easily and turn the film black. Different tissues within the body let different amounts of X-rays through and, all together, give us a picture of what is going on inside. I was expecting to see a collection of party-popper-shaped objects inside the greedy dog's stomach. Because plastic doesn't show up very well on a radiograph, they would not be as obvious as a stone or a metal ring would, but I felt sure I would be able to see them outlined by the other contents of the stomach. Jelly and sausage rolls do not show up at all because, on an X-ray at least, they look just the same as liver, spleen or intestines.

Not so long ago I saw a radiograph of the stomach of a dog who had eaten some plastic ducks, like the ones that float in a child's bath. They were very clear on the image, which looked pretty funny. But, today, I could not see any shapes that looked like whole party poppers. This had to mean that Quercus had chewed them into pieces of plastic, lengths of stringy confetti and gunpowder mixed in there too. I did not need to operate, but I was worried about the powder mixing with the stomach acid. I couldn't see the cufflinks in there either.

What to do?

After a lengthy discussion with the rest of the team, we concluded that we should wake Quercus up by reversing his sedation, and then try to make him sick so that the dangerous chemicals, any nasty sharp bits of plastic and the stringy confetti would come back up rather than continuing down through his small intestines, where they could cause other serious problems.

I called Sandra, who was very relieved that their big, hairy dog would not need an operation. But, of all the things I have to do as a veterinary surgeon, making a dog sick is my *least favourite*. I would rather empty anal glands or even clean up poo. Vets spend much of their time trying to *stop* dogs and cats from being sick, or feeling sick. But now I would be deliberately making Quercus feel awful – really awful. So awful, in fact, that he would vomit up all of his stomach contents.

I knelt beside the big, grey and by now very confused hound.

'I'm really sorry, Quercus,' I said. I felt I should offer him some explanation. 'I'm going to give you another injection, but it won't make you feel better. In fact, it will make you feel worse. You'll start gulping, you'll feel worried and a sad and anxious expression will appear on your face. Then you'll look at me and, if you could talk, you'd say, "Gosh, I feel awful." Then you'll vomit three times if you're lucky, or five times if you're unlucky. But after that you will feel much better and there will be three or five piles of vomit, hopefully containing party popper bits and maybe even the elusive cufflinks. You will feel a little bit sick for a while but at least you won't need an operation and at least you won't explode. Is that okay?'

Quercus had no idea what I was talking about.

I gave him the tiny injection and waited for the worried expression to appear across his confused face. It did, quickly followed by the gulping and a new expression of deepening concern and deeper confusion. I held his enormous ears out of the way so he wasn't sick on them, which would have been the final insult.

Then poor Quercus started to heave. Out came pieces of plastic, streamers, bits of paper packaging, mangled balloons and some suspicious, grey sludge that looked like gunpowder mixed with stomach acid. Several piles of chewed-up party apparatus appeared before he stopped looking worried and started to wag his tail again. Quickly, I took him back to his kennel – the daft dog had started sniffing the vomit and I thought he was about to eat it again.

Quercus, though he had been sick several times and still felt groggy, was a lucky pup. He would make a full recovery. I phoned Sandra with news of the afternoon's activities and the outlook for him.

Jonathon and Sandra were soon back at the surgery to collect their beloved but rather naughty dog.

'Goodbye Quercus,' I called as he trotted out to the car. 'I'm sorry I made you sick but I'm happy you didn't explode. Oh, and have a good party, Jonathon!'

As young Quercus, now happily sitting in the back seat of the car, looked at me from under his hairy eyebrows, I felt sure that this would not be the last time we met.

I never did hear if the cufflinks turned up.

19. Husband and Wife Save an Alpaca and Other Animals

I t was a grey day in November and I needed some help to operate on an alpaca. Jackie, the alpaca farmer with whom I work a great deal, was looking after an alpaca for a friend. The elderly old alpaca girl, jet black in colour, was appropriately called Ebony. Jackie had called me out the week before, worried about a mass on Ebony's foot that had been growing steadily for a few months. It immediately caused me some concern. It was the size of a small apple, firm, irregular and extending around the outer toe, below the fetlock on the hind leg. Given its position and nature, it really needed to be removed as soon as possible. What I wouldn't know until I started operating was whether the mass was removable on its own or whether the whole toe would have to be amputated. It was not your usual type of surgery and it was sure to be a challenge. My plan was to sedate Ebony deeply so that she lay down and stayed still for the duration. I would administer some local anaesthetic to the foot to numb the area. I'd also need to be quick and efficient with my surgery; if the alpaca woke up prematurely, the operation would be a disaster. I was keen to have another set of professional eyes to help me make the right decision on this nasty, sarcomatous mass. (Sarcomatous refers to a type of tumour called a 'sarcoma'. These are nasty and aggressive and, although they do not necessarily spread, you do not want a sarcomatous tumour.) Another pair of hands would make the procedure much quicker. As I arranged the visit with Jackie, I searched for a veterinary volunteer to help me. As usual when difficult procedures on a peculiar animal are concerned, everyone was suddenly very busy and looked in the opposite direction, but Anne, always up for a new challenge, offered to come along to help.

Anne and I had been working together again since I joined the practice in Boroughbridge, where she was already working part-time as well as holding down another job at a different practice. Experienced vets are hard to come by and her skills and experience were in demand. It was nice to be professional colleagues again, mainly because we worked well together, but also because it brought back memories of the many occasions at the beginning of our careers when we had helped one another out, as vets or vets-to-be.

At vet school, Anne was in the year above me and I'd often help out when she did her shifts on night duty. 'Hut duty', as it was called, was a full week on call, staying at the vet school to help with inpatients and emergencies. I think it got the name because, historically, students who were on call slept in a small hut at the school. By the time we arrived there was a flat above the clinic for the purpose, but the name had stuck. We had to do three week-long stints during our final year and they were very hard work, involving multiple night-time checks at best and at worst no sleep at all. This was in addition to the already heavy daytime caseload. I think it has changed now, partly because it took many students to the edge of exhaustion and sanity, but in the mid-1990s 'hut duties' were there to be endured rather than enjoyed. So, because I was a keen student and because I loved being immersed in the clinical action, I used to try to spend those weeks with Anne in the little flat next to the veterinary hospital. I'm not sure if I was supposed to be there, since I was in my penultimate year and not fully equipped with all the skills to help, but I loved it and the clinicians – some of whom I was getting to know quite well – didn't seem to mind. It seemed that everyone welcomed an extra pair of hands.

I remember late on one of the first evenings of Anne's hut duty, a dog was suffering some kind of crisis and there was a new clinician in charge, fresh from his PhD. He was flapping around (literally – his unbuttoned white coat was flailing around the prep room as he dashed about), trying to work out what to do with the dog. Knowledgeable as he was in the theory of canine hormonal diseases, the novice veterinary surgeon was new to this kind of emergency work and seemed somewhat lacking in clinical experience. I tried to look inconspicuous as Anne and two of her fellow final-year students hovered nervously, awaiting guidance from the more senior vet, who was getting into more and more of a tizz as the crisis deepened. He was struggling to know what to do next, and began to panic.

'Well it might be helpful if you stopped shouting at us!' Anne blurted out, exasperated. 'You are supposed to be showing us what to do.' Everyone froze – you weren't supposed to speak to a clinician like that. In my mind, from my corner of the kennels I came to the rescue, offering exactly the correct test and the right sized catheter to save the day. In reality, one of the students got the head of department on the phone and the poor dog eventually received the correct care and everything ended well. After that occasion, I became more useful, taking the temperatures of sick calves and injecting the various medications. Helpful or not, what stuck in my mind was how exciting it was for Anne and me to be working together as trainee vets.

Once Anne had qualified, I was a useful companion again, as her first year in practice coincided with my final year at vet school. When she wasn't on duty, Anne would drive back up to Cambridge, happy to spend more time in that beautiful place where we were privileged to have studied. On the weekends she was working, my little red Metro and I would make the journey to her flat in Hampshire. The flat was the annexe to a big house, miles away from anywhere, up a tiny lane in the middle of the countryside. It was a lovely flat but very remote, and it typified the isolation that many vets encounter during their first job in practice, a long way from the hustle and bustle and supercharged social atmosphere of vet school. Luckily for Anne, she was on home turf and had friends and family nearby. I was always happy to visit and loved helping out with calls or with hospitalised patients. The worst thing about staying when Anne was on duty was the huge, cream-coloured Bakelite telephone, which resided next to the bed. Its ring was so loud that it was probably heard in the next village. There was no chance of sleeping through a night-time call, but a reasonable chance of having a heart attack before even leaving the house!

In the summer of 1996, after I'd graduated and started my job in Thirsk, Anne searched for a mixed-practice post somewhere nearby. But to find the perfect mixed practice job, with the right balance of work and close enough to Thirsk to manage when on call, proved to be almost impossible. She scoured the *Veterinary Record* every week until, finally, an advert appeared seeking a vet for a practice in Bedale, which was only about ten miles away. It sounded ideal. Bedale was a lovely town on the edge of the Yorkshire Dales that promised the Herriotesque work that we all strived for, and Anne, up in Thirsk for the weekend, quickly picked up the phone to arrange an interview. However, it wasn't long before she appeared back in the sitting room looking bewildered and frustrated.

'Any luck?' I enquired, sensing all had not gone to plan.

'It's no good, I'm afraid,' she said, shaking her head. 'Back to the drawing board. I asked about the job, but before I could even say anything else, and I still can't quite believe this actually happened, the senior partner said: "We've always found it better to employ male vets. They cope better with the farm work."'

Incredulous at the undisguised prejudice, she went on: 'I was so surprised I just said, "Oh, okay, thank you very much" and that was the end of the conversation!'

Even in the late 1990s this was obviously not an acceptable thing to think, let alone say out loud! Anne was furious and would have refused the job even had an offer been forthcoming. This misogynistic attitude was, unfortunately, all too common in the profession at that time. Thankfully, such overt discrimination in the veterinary world is now in large part a thing of the past, but I suspect this has been driven more by necessity than proper 'egality'. Even in the last few years, I've been sadly disappointed by the persistence of prejudice within older members of my profession, and it still has a corrosive influence. Things will improve when the 'old-school' vets have finally all retired. At least, I hope things will improve. If not, then there is no future for our profession.

So, there was to be no job for Anne in Yorkshire, at least not for the time being. She quickly got a wonderful job in the Cotswolds, in a picturesque town called Broadway. It was, in many ways, idyllic. Idyllic, but three and a half hours from where I lived and worked in North Yorkshire. By now, the rota issue was playing havoc with our free time. Anne was working two out of five weekends and I was working one weekend in two. It doesn't take a mathematician to work out that this gave us nearly no time off together, so we were back to helping each other out on our free weekends. If Anne was working and I was off, I went to stay in the Cotswolds; if Anne was off, she would come to see me in Yorkshire. This allowed us more time together, but practically no time off together *and* away from vet action. It was a pain in the neck, but one to which we eventually became habituated, at least to some extent. Working together was still fun though, and I got to know the area around Cheltenham, Winchcombe and Broadway very well, even becoming acquainted with some of the farmers. The other vets in the practice loved it when I came to stay, because they knew that their second on call would be quiet; I was on hand to step in and accompany my girlfriend to the practice and to farms.

'I owe Julian a bottle of wine for helping out with that cow's Caesar on Saturday night,' was a frequent start to conversation on a Monday morning when Anne returned to work after a busy weekend on call. In reality, it meant that there was almost never any escape from the beeper, either in my pocket in Yorkshire, or Anne's pocket in the Cotswolds.

The first occasion on which this happened was particularly memorable. Thankfully, the Bakelite telephone had been left in Hampshire so there was no heart-attack-inducing 'ring-ring' to wrench us from our sleep, but it was cold, dark and one o'clock in the morning. A cow was struggling to calve and the farmer, who had a large herd on the edge of the escarpment above the picturesque village of Snowshill, knew she needed a Caesarean section.

'It's at Hannay's,' Anne explained, although this meant nothing to me.

'It's a big suckler herd. I've been there before and they have a good herd. They are good farmers too, so if they need a vet to help calve a cow, it's sure to be a tough one.'

I couldn't stay in bed – I'd need to go and help but while it was certainly an inconvenience on what should have been my weekend off, it wasn't actually *my* beeper and it wasn't *my* call, so it wouldn't be me feeling the pressure or making decisions.

I sat in the passenger seat and enjoyed the nocturnal journey. An on-call vet sees all sorts of interesting things while driving down deserted lanes at night – owls silently flying across moonlit fields or sitting on gateposts, deer, picked out by the headlights, cantering across the road, foxes getting on with their duties. However, the nausea inherent in being suddenly wrenched from sleep, along with the anxiety over what might be in store with the patient, means that seldom does this bring quite the joy that it should. But on this evening, as passenger and assistant, I got a great thrill from seeing the wonderful wildlife of the British night, and exclaimed at the magnificence of it all. Anne was less excited, facing the prospect of some difficult work ahead – it was, after all, her responsibility to get the calf out!

There was an awkward introduction when we arrived on the farm. The farmer knew Anne, although not very well (I think she'd been there just once or twice before), and seemed surprised to see me.

'This is Julian, my boyfriend. He's staying this weekend,' Anne introduced me as we made our way across the yard. 'He's a vet, so he knows what he's doing. I'm hoping he might help, if that's all right with you? At least it saves waking up my boss.' Anne tried to make light of the slightly embarrassing situation.

In the gloom of the cowshed, Anne felt inside the cow to assess the chances of the calf being delivered normally. She quickly conceded that surgery would be necessary. I was glad she didn't canvass my opinion, which some vets would have done to confirm the decision. My role was mainly to help to get the cow and the equipment ready for the op, not to make clinical judgements. I assumed my position to help pull the calf out of the cow's uterus. This is really the purpose of a helper when doing a cow Caesarean. It's really quite hard to do the operation single-handed and relies on everything going according to plan. Nowadays, I do try to do most of my cow Caesars on my own, mainly to save disturbing the second on-call vet in the small hours, but at the start of a vet's career it is important to have another pair of professional hands. I scrubbed my arms and plunged them down next to Anne's into the depths of the bovine abdomen. We lifted the heavy uterus up and I held it in place, just outside the long, vertical incision she'd made in the cow's left flank. Anne carefully cut through the muscular wall of the uterus and I grabbed first one, then the other of the calf's back legs and between us we pulled the calf out into a frosty world. Cold air surged into its lungs and the huge calf spluttered into life, coughing the mucus from its lungs. We knew it would be fine. The next job was the suturing. Anne placed the sutures and I cut them off – first catgut for the uterus, then more catgut for the muscle layers and finally thick nylon sutures for the skin.

It was nearly three in the morning by the time we had finished, but our first nocturnal veterinary adventure had gone smoothly. It had been a slick and efficient night's work if ever there had been one and the farmer, happy with our work and the outcome, invited us into the farmhouse for a cup of coffee. We chatted for another hour. It had been a good night, successful, hard and physical farm work, and it had been irrelevant whether the surgeon was in possession of two X chromosomes or an X and a Y. Bedale's loss was Broadway's gain. But, hey, that's misogyny and prejudice for you! It doesn't get you very far.

So, twenty-two years later, driving up to the village of Husthwaite together to see Ebony brought back memories for us both of that time at Hannay's farm in the Cotswolds. This time it was me driving and it was daytime rather than the depths of night. The call was less urgent too, but no less stressful for the surgeon. The operation would be a tough one and I needed Anne's help, both to ensure the sedation was smooth and also to give another clinical opinion. It was good to be working together again.

As we clambered out of the car to meet Jackie and Ebony, there was an added challenge to be overcome, beyond the surgical procedure and managing the sedation. It was not one that either of us would have ever envisaged twenty-odd years ago as we slurped our coffee in the early hours at Hannay's farm.

'Morning Julian, hello Anne,' said Ross excitedly as he emerged from the alpaca shed with a camera on his shoulder. 'How are you feeling about the operation? What are you worried about? What are the challenges facing the two of you today?'

Ross was my current producer-director. He had already been at the farm for half an hour, getting ready to film our operation for *The Yorkshire Vet*. He pointed his camera at the pair of us, waiting for an engaging response from either Anne or me. I felt like apologising to Anne for the situation we now found ourselves in. It was a million miles from that early morning in the farmer's kitchen, when life was simple, in the days before television scrutiny. Days when we were younger, and free.

20. Terrible Tumours

I had not seen Rodney for a while. Lambing time was long finished and the farmer, who lived quite close to my hometown of Castleford in West Yorkshire, was enjoying the relaxing part of the sheep farmer's year. The long summer days made life easier than the cold, damp darkness that characterised the early-morning lambing checks and late-night shifts necessary to supervise his beloved flock throughout the spring. As well as the sheep and goats upon which he doted, Rodney also had a family of Border collies. I say a family, because many of his dogs were actually related – mothers, fathers, brothers, sisters and aunts – and they all had similar and endearing characters. They were also part of *his* family.

During the summer, when the sheep looked after themselves, Rodney turned his attention to training his newest sheepdog. It was a matter of great pride to him that he should do it himself and do it well. Luckily, his training technique involved the younger dogs learning the ropes from their more accomplished, older relatives. I had seen this first-hand on a couple of occasions when I'd called in to see Rodney, often on my way back to North Yorkshire after a visit to see my parents in Castleford or my sister in Leeds. He would use a small group of experienced ewes, ones that knew which way to trot and which way to go around the field. These sheep almost steered themselves around the gates and obstacles in the gently sloping paddock behind the sheep shed and around the pond. One or two of his older dogs – Milly or Jet, for example – would go out with Flynn, the youngest of the trainees. Rodney would teach and the older dogs would guide and nudge and the younger dog would learn. This meant that there was always a job for the old dogs on Rodney's farm, whereas some farmers, working the bigger hills or the more exposed moors of rugged North Yorkshire, would have put their old collies into retirement if their aching joints could no longer cope with hard duties on the fell.

But the mentoring process wasn't the only reason Rodney wanted the best for all his dogs. As well as recognising their importance to him as teachers, he loved them. On one occasion, he told me, tongue in cheek (I think) and in the broadest of Wakefield accents, 'More than me wife, you know, if truth be told.'

The first dog of Rodney's that I had the privilege to treat was his old favourite, Milly. She had a tumour in her mouth. It was an acanthomatous ameloblastoma, which was as nasty as it sounded – an aggressive tumour, invading the bone of her lower jaw. Mercifully it was not one that would spread around her body, but, nevertheless, it would destroy and take over her face and, if not addressed quickly, would bring an early end to her life. The local vet Rodney had seen near to his home had said the prognosis was terrible and there was nothing to be done: Milly would have to be put to sleep. Rodney could not bring himself to give up on the elderly collie and so he came to see me for a second opinion.

I decided to try to remove the mass, along with part of Milly's lower jaw – not surgery for the faint-hearted. It went as well as I could have hoped and Rodney was as grateful as anyone I had ever seen.

Today, Milly came along with Rodney and Jet, the latest of the problematic collies from West Yorkshire. It was nice to see her, with her wagging tail at one end and happy, smiling face at the other, still going strong three years after the op.

'I'm worried, Julian,' Rodney explained. 'This is Jet, Milly's mum.' Jet was Rodney's oldest collie, and she and Milly were chips off the same block. The two dogs sat next to me, nuzzling their noses against my face, as he went on to describe the problem.

'She has a lump on her side. I noticed it last week and it's quite big. I'm just not raight 'appy abart it. It dunt look right, so I thought I'd best bring her to see yer,' and then to Jet, 'Get over on yer side, Jet. Let Julian 'ave a look.' And with that Jet rolled over, without even the slightest hesitation, such was her complete trust in Rodney.

The lump was evident, though it wasn't on her side. Jet had a mammary tumour. It was knobbly, hard and the size of a large tangerine, and cause for serious concern. Mammary cancers are nasty things, in dogs as in people, and the presence of such a lump is always a problem. The fact that Rodney had only noticed it a week ago, and that it was now a considerable size, indicated another reason to be worried – it had grown quickly. Mammary tumours are the most common type of cancer in dogs. They are much less common in spayed bitches – which is one of the reasons vets recommend females be neutered – and rare in male dogs. They take various forms, but the commonest type starts off as a benign growth and then changes its characteristics to become a mixed carcinoma. Removal at the earliest opportunity is always the best course of action.

I discussed with Rodney what to do. Although he was clearly anxious about the future of his geriatric collie, the matriarch of his collection, I hadn't let him down so far with my care of his animals and he agreed to leave Jet with me, for surgery the following morning. Rodney waved her goodbye and Jet settled in for bed, no breakfast to come but at least an evening meal to gobble up.

Jet was first on my list the next day. The first thing to do was to take some chest X-rays to check for metastases – secondary tumours that might have already spread to the lungs. In cases like this, where the mass has appeared over just a short space of time, it may not have had time to spread and, even if has, the secondaries can be too small to show up on an X-ray. However, it is important to check, as there is little to be gained from invasive surgery to remove a mammary mass if there is a big tumour or tumours in the lungs. Thankfully, Jet's chest X-rays were clear and it wasn't long before she was fully anaesthetised, clipped and prepped, ready to go.

I love surgery. It is an instant way to relieve a problem. To remove a tumour, suture a wound, screw together a broken bone to stabilise a fracture or add an artificial ligament to repair a disrupted joint provides an instant solution to the patient's problem. It is very satisfying, but also challenging. Before every cut, the outcome and the next step must be considered. Today, it was crucial that Jet's tumour came out in its entirety. If any tumour cells were left behind it would quickly regrow. I had to make sure the edges of her skin came together, neatly and without any tension that could hamper the healing. I needed to quell the flow of blood that pumps from an artery. There were some big arteries in this area, which would squirt rhythmically and insistently if not clamped and then ligated efficiently. And I needed to decide whether to insert a drain – a soft rubber tube – to prevent a build-up of fluid in the space under the skin left after the tumour had been removed.

My mind, during surgery like this, is full of surgical thoughts, constantly calculating and recalculating, while also keeping at least half an eye out to make sure the nurse is happy with the anaesthetic, especially in an elderly patient like Jet. Surgery in first-opinion veterinary practice is very much an exercise in multi-tasking. This is okay, though. I'm quite good at multitasking.

Before long, Jet's mammary tumour was sitting in a pot of formalin, safely resected from the surrounding tissue. The vessels were tied off and the subcutaneous tissue apposed, and only a long row of nylon sutures marked the place where the mass had once been. I turned off the gas and rolled Jet onto her side, allowing the stoic old dog to wake up slowly. Once she had lifted her head it was time to make the phone call that Rodney had been awaiting.

'Morning Rodney. All good news here,' I reported. 'Jet's done very well, she's sitting up and I think we've got all of her tumour out. She should be good to go home later this afternoon. She's done very well.'

'Thank you, Julian. I knew she'd be raight. You've never let me down yet. I'll be up at abart fouwer to get her.' And that, as far as Rodney was concerned, was that. As I went back to the kennels to check on Jet's recovery, I thought about all the other times over the years that I had watched over members of her family under my care. It was a lovely feeling. And of course, Rodney would be here soon – just after four o'clock.

It wasn't long before I encountered another doting owner, just as anxious about her dog. I had not met Mrs Liddle before, but we had a mutual friend, known by most people who knew her as 'Auntie Julie'.

Julie has a boarding kennels just outside Thirsk, and I have looked after both her boarders and her own dogs for many years. Our own dog, Emmy, goes to stay with Auntie Julie when we are on holiday and she loves it (although she has generally sneaked into the house to share a dog bed with her best friend, Julie's Jack Russell Titch, rather than slumming it in one of the luxury kennels!). Many years ago, before starting her boarding kennels, Julie worked as a veterinary nurse at the surgery in Boroughbridge, where I work now. What she doesn't know about dogs, their habits and their traits isn't worth knowing.

After a recent stay in her kennels, Julie had recommended that Mrs Liddle bring her dog, a little West Highland White Terrier called Duffy, to see me. Julie had noticed that he wasn't quite as little as he had been the last time he had stayed with her, and didn't feel he was quite his normal self.

'You should take him to see Julian,' she advised, 'I think his tummy is getting bigger and it would be worth getting it checked.'

Within a week, Mrs Liddle and her fluffy dog were in the waiting room. By strange coincidence it was the same day that Jet was in to have her stitches removed. As the two dogs' paths crossed in the waiting room, one having finished her treatment and the other, as yet, undiagnosed, none of us could have imagined that they would be contiguous and slightly connected stories in a book!

Mrs Liddle had been somewhat dissatisfied by the service she had received at her former vets, where excessive, extensive and expensive tests had proved more of a hindrance than a help in diagnosing previous problems. Based on Julie's recommendation, she'd sought me out instead and now here she was, rubbing shoulders with Rodney. While the elegant, elderly lady's clipped tones were very different from Rodney's broad West Yorkshire,

they shared a deep devotion to their dogs and a loving but pragmatic approach to their care.

'Hello, Julian, I'm so glad I've been able to see you today.'
Mrs Liddle greeted me enthusiastically as I called her into the
consulting room. 'Thank you for fitting me in. I know you are
very busy. Julie speaks *very* highly of you. She is a bit of a fan,
I think!'

I knew straight away that Mrs Liddle would be crystal clear
in her summary of the little dog's signs. Sometimes, it is hard
to pick out the salient details from a pet's history. Not today
though. Mrs Liddle gave a succinct and accurate explanation of
the problem.

'Well. It's his tummy. I think it's getting bigger. He does eat
plenty – my husband likes to give him treats – but I just think,
really and truly, it is *too* big. What do you think?'

I lifted the rotund Westie onto my consulting room table and
peered at his abdomen. It did look bigger than it should. There
were a number of possible causes so, rather than focusing on
the area in question straight away, I started my examination at
his head and worked back. Everything forward of his distended
abdomen was okay, but the abdomen itself most definitely was
not.

'My word, he is pretty big, isn't he?' I agreed, trying not to
sound rude or to express too much concern at this early stage.

'Well, yes. *Could* it be too much food, like my husband says?
Or do you think it's . . .' Mrs Liddle paused for a moment, before
leaning across the Westie and the table and continuing in a
hushed tone, '. . . something more serious?'

It was obvious that something was wrong, but I tried not to
change my facial expression or make any of those noises that a
concerned builder makes before pronouncing how difficult a job
might be.

'You were right to bring him, Mrs Liddle,' I assured her, cautiously. 'I think Duffy may have a mass of some kind. We'll need to do some X-rays, an ultrasound scan and some blood tests to help us find out what it is.'

I didn't want to cause too much alarm but I was fairly certain the situation was serious.

'Can you leave him with us this afternoon? We'll get on with it all straight away.'

I was keen to get a diagnosis as promptly as I could.

Sure enough, the imaging confirmed my fears – Duffy had an enormous tumour in the front part of his abdomen. I called Mrs Liddle with the bad news and she returned to the surgery straight away so that we could discuss the options. It was likely that the mass was on either the spleen (which would be less bad) or on the liver (which would be very bad). A splenic mass could be removed fairly easily, but if the mass was in the liver surgical removal would be very difficult or impossible. I could take biopsies to confirm the origin of the tumour, either through the skin or by doing exploratory surgery. Exploratory surgery would give me the option to remove the growth if it was amenable, and would also allow me to see if it had already spread to other parts of the abdomen. Sadly, if this was the case, the prognosis was likely to be hopeless. I also explained that euthanasia was another option. Some owners would take this route, not through pessimism, but because of an unwillingness to let their dog undergo invasive surgery in the light of a grave prognosis.

Mrs Liddle nodded and pulled faces in agreement and disagreement at different parts of our discussion, and we quickly agreed that the best course of action was to put Duffy under anaesthetic and perform an exploratory laparotomy. Mrs Liddle wanted me to do everything I could, as long as it was the best for Duffy. By now, however, evening surgery was about to start.

It was likely to be a big op, and I thought I would probably need an extra pair of hands. I knew Anne was in the following morning and would be happy to help.

'Can you bring him back in the morning?' I asked. This would give me a bit of time to plan the procedure. It would also give Mrs Liddle an evening to come to terms with the news – an evening that could well be her last with little Duffy. If the growth was inoperable, then Duffy might not be coming around from his anaesthetic.

'Of course, Julian.' She nodded bravely. 'What time would you like him?'

'Half past eight would be perfect.' I tried to sound reassuring. 'I'll see you tomorrow. And remember, no breakfast.' Had the distension in Duffy's abdomen been just fat and not a terrible tumour, my advice about breakfast might still have been the same.

It wasn't just Duffy who went without breakfast the following morning. I was worried about what I might find and had no appetite for food. I talked the case over with Anne, who was calmly reassuring. Between the two of us we would be able to work out the best course of action for the little dog. We'd do everything we could.

By half past nine Duffy was asleep, lying in the most undignified of positions, on his back with the whole of his abdomen shaved. He looked like a turkey ready for the oven. I took hold of my scalpel, took a deep breath and made the incision through the body wall and into his abdominal cavity. The mass, which we had known was big, was even bigger once it was visible. I extended the incision so that I could see the full extent of the situation and gently felt under the lump, easing it to the surface and then carefully nudging it out of the abdomen.

'Bugger,' and other words beginning with 'B' came out of the mouths of everyone nearby. The enormous mass was attached to poor Duffy's liver. I'd never seen such a huge lump on a dog's liver before. Usually renal tumours cause serious illness before they reach such a massive size and my first reaction was to reach for the telephone to make the sad call. However, as I explored the rest of the abdomen, two things became apparent. One was that there were no signs of spread. This was, at least, one small positive. The other was that the mass seemed to be confined to just one lobe of the liver, while the other lobes all looked normal. The anaesthetic was stable, and while Duffy was big he was not too poorly. Surely two more good things. As I explored further, I looked to Anne for some reassurance. Then I looked to everyone else in theatre for reassurance. Not much was forthcoming.

Then I made a snap decision.

'I'm going to remove this,' I announced, without really thinking how I would manage to do it. 'If I can remove this whole liver lobe, I'll get all of the tumour out. I just need to go across there.'

Buoyed with a huge surge of possibly misplaced optimism, I pointed my forceps at the base of the tumour.

'What do you think?' I looked at Anne. She didn't look convinced.

'I suppose if we can get right under there and tie it all off, we might be able to do it,' she conceded. 'Okay, let's give it a go.'

So, the two of us set about removing the biggest liver tumour either of us had ever seen and, to cut a long surgical story short, Duffy woke up from his anaesthetic considerably slimmer and a bit sore, but otherwise remarkably unperturbed by the whole experience.

The following day he went home, almost as if nothing had happened. The brave little terrier trotted out into the waiting room and Mrs Liddle gave me the biggest hug.

'Thank you, Julian. I really do think this has been a miracle!'

As well as a hug and an emotional vote of thanks, she also gave me a huge cigar and a bottle of Burgundy. I didn't need any presents – treating Duffy had been the biggest reward of all. Watching him walk cheerfully out of the door and seeing the relief in his owner's face was all I needed to make this a brilliant day. Although, the bottle of Burgundy did turn out to be something rather special.

21. Grateful Owners, Unusual Gifts

As soon as Mrs Liddle handed me that bottle of wine I knew it was something to be cherished. It was a 2000 premier cru Burgundy. I tend not to drink Burgundy, because the Pinot Noir grape from which it derives is too light for my taste (or at least, all those I had drunk up until this point had been). Give me a hefty Bordeaux, Côtes du Rhône or a decent Malbec any time. However, I am interested in wine and this bottle intrigued me. I don't know nearly as much as I would like to, so I took a photo of the bottle before stowing it in the wine rack in the kitchen at home, intending to do some research. Amusingly, beside it was a bottle I had won in a raffle the previous weekend – and that was the full extent of my current wine collection. Having just two bottles of wine in the house constituted, in my mind, a minor emergency – what if friends arrived, unannounced, for an impromptu party?

Anne was quick to point out that firstly, this was very unlikely and secondly, if more than two bottles' worth of guests arrived out of the blue, Tesco was only five minutes away. Therefore, it was not strictly necessary to have two cases of wine in reserve at all times. Nevertheless, I was perturbed not to be prepared for this possible emergency so, the following Saturday after I'd finished morning surgery, I walked down to the local wine shop in Boroughbridge to replenish my depleted supplies. Nick, who owned the shop, was a font of wine knowledge and was always happy to open a bottle to try, which made Saturday a better time for me to visit him than during a busy week. As I perused his shelves, I told him about the bottle and showed him the photo on my phone.

'Ah, very nice indeed.' He nodded, 'A 2000 Vosne Romanée, Aux Reignots. It's one of Sylvain Cathiard's. That's a good one. I'll look it up in my book and find you some details.' He reached for a Bible-like book, itself almost as big as a case of wine.

As I continued my search for moderately priced bottles to fill the spaces in my wine rack at home, Nick, engrossed in his massive book, started to show signs of bewilderment.

'This is very strange. Your wine is not in my book. I've never had this happen before. It must be a rare one. *All* wine is in my book.'

He asked to scrutinise my photo again, before screwing up his face and pushing his glasses up onto his forehead as if that would help him to find information that wasn't there.

'Hmm. I definitely can't find it. This is unusual. I'll do some research and get back to you.'

We exchanged email addresses.

'What should I do with it?' I asked. 'I don't really like Burgundy – I always think it's a bit watery. If it's a good one, surely it will be wasted on me?'

'Not at all! You must drink it. No question about it. You'll need to drink it with some partridge, or possibly guinea fowl. Let me find out some details though. It's very interesting.' Nick's grin, which was growing bigger and bigger, told me just how excited he was about the rarity of the bottle in question. I didn't tell him that it was sitting next to a bottle that still had a raffle ticket taped to its screw top.

'If Burgundy is not your thing, what you need to do is *train* your taste buds,' Nick went on, clearly having spotted a sales opportunity. 'Burgundy is an acquired taste. You need to work up to a bottle like that. Here, try this,' he continued enthusiastically, as he pulled various bottles of wine from the shelves, regaling me with the details of each one.

'Drink this at the weekend and see what you think. And then next week we can move onto the league above.'

I could see where this was going, but I offered only limited resistance and left the shop with some moderately expensive wine under my arm – some to fill my wine rack and a bottle of entry-level Burgundy to start the education of my palate. The gift from Duffy's owner was a cracker and I was very grateful and very excited, as it appeared to be opening up a whole new chapter in my wine drinking. I have received a fair few thank-you gifts over my career, but this bottle appeared, at least so far, to be the most interesting.

Towards the end of my university course, we were all subjected to some lectures about financial planning and running a veterinary business. Not many of us were particularly engaged with these topics – we just wanted to get out there and practise. It became a standing joke that I had declared: 'I'd be happy to do the job for a sack of potatoes.' Of course there was some flippancy in my claim, but it reflected the fact that I was (as were we all) following this career path for the genuine love of animals and total dedication to our vocation rather than for any outright financial gain. Clearly this was naïve and, after my first year or so in practice, my philosophy would come back to haunt me, particularly because to receive a bag of potatoes from a farmer would *actually* help the financial hardship that most young veterinary graduates faced. We worked incredibly long hours for not much money. My first salary was fourteen thousand pounds a year, for working seventy or eighty hours or more each week with just four weeks holiday. A sack of potatoes if a farmer was grateful for a successful lambing was a very welcome boost.

Brian Bentley from Old Byland, a traditional Yorkshire farmer if ever there was one, would always offer me a pair of swedes after I had tended to his cattle or sheep up in the wilds of the moors. The first time he offered me some of the tough vegetables, I misheard him.

'Do you like swedes?' he muttered, stomping off in the direction of one of the sheds. I thought he said 'sweets'.

'I do, yes. I love them,' I called after him. 'They are great on a busy day when I've missed my lunch. They give me an instant rush of energy. Especially chocolate, but I'm not fussy.'

Brian hadn't heard the second part of my reply, as he'd disappeared into the shed. He emerged a moment later with an armful of mud-encrusted swedes, which would require a good deal of time and effort before I could extract any energy from their wholesome flesh. As it happens, I *do* like swedes as well as sweets, but Brian never seemed to remember that he had asked me before, so at the end of every visit came the same question: 'Do you like swedes?' I'd always reply in the affirmative, and, as I left the farm with a couple of the rock-hard vegetables rolling around in my footwell, I used to laugh and recall my excitement at the offer of some of the farmer's confectionery.

Over the years, I have got to know many rather eccentric but always fascinating elderly ladies. They seem to enjoy the company of an enthusiastic young vet, and in return offer sage pieces of advice and worldly wisdom. On several occasions, they have also shared old trinkets, which can sometimes be nice and are always memorable!

Mrs G. was a great friend, a wise advisor when it came to old-fashioned medical techniques and tricks and, on at least a couple of occasions, someone with whom I spent an evening drinking cocktails. Her expertise in mixing cocktails was honed during her youth, when her family dominated the trading routes around the sea ports of the British Empire. One of these evenings was a thank-you for treating her favourite and faithful old Labrador, affectionately known as Fish Face. I do not know why he was called Fish Face, because he neither looked nor smelt like a fish, but that is how everyone knew him. I had looked after him for many years, performed the honours at the end of his long life and even helped to dig the hole where he was finally to be laid to rest.

However, the gift I remembered most fondly from Mrs G. was not one of the evenings enjoying Singapore Slings, but a small, brown, slightly stained bottle of a mysterious medicine called Friar's Balsam. I can't remember its exact purpose, but I do remember Mrs G. being obsessed by its fantastic healing properties (for nearly all conditions) and her great frustration at its dwindling availability. The Veterinary Medicine Directorate or the National Institute for Health and Care Excellence must have declared the miracle drug obsolete; but Mrs G. was still managing to procure, from somewhere, the elixir. I imagined it coming from the depths of some camphor-lined trunk covered with luggage labels from the Punjab, Cape Town or the East India Company – it certainly hadn't come from Boots the Chemist. At least, not in the last fifty years.

I thanked Mrs G. for the generous gift and placed the

sought-after tonic on the shelf in my consulting room. I wasn't convinced it would be the first drug I would reach for in my medicinal armoury, but it was a kind and thoughtful gesture.

One gift that was most definitely NOT useless arrived in a package one day while I was working in Thirsk, shortly after the airing of series two of *The Yorkshire Vet*. One of the episodes had shown my former colleague Peter Wright and myself lamenting the demise of the mercury thermometer in favour of its digital successor. While these devices are modern and clinical, they are prone to running out of batteries, they beep in an annoying way and it remains a mystery to me how to change the scale between Celsius and Fahrenheit. Good old-fashioned mercury thermometers, while they might upset the Health and Safety Executive (glass is sharp if it breaks and mercury is bad for people), do not beep annoyingly, they never run out of batteries and they have both Celsius and Fahrenheit scales. The reading can be translated both by old-fashioned farmers who have never heard of Celsius and millennials who have never heard of Fahrenheit. They are very useful pieces of kit, albeit rather old-fashioned.

The glass thermometers are increasingly hard to find, but a few days after the episode in question, the brown paper package was delivered, addressed to me and 'HANDLE WITH CARE' written in big, scrawled letters on the outside. I opened it with trepidation to find it crammed full of ancient glass thermometers, each held in a neat metal tube. They had come from a retired nurse, anxious for her old-fashioned tools to be put to good use on any patient, be they human or otherwise. They were from a similar era to the Friar's Balsam, but immeasurably more practical. I'm still using them today and I smile every time I unscrew the metal cap to retrieve one of them from its case.

Another colourful elderly lady, of whom I became very fond, was Mrs Taylor. She kept guinea pigs, which she loved and which

I visited occasionally, but her biggest loves were her dogs, Mitzi, an ancient but energetic poodle, and Billy, a lackadaisical Shih-Tzu. Mitzi was in super health, defiant of her age, but Billy had a multitude of minor problems, which meant I treated him regularly. His main ailment arose from his enthusiasm for Mrs Taylor's tasty and wholesome meals-on-wheels, which were delivered to her home every day. Mrs Taylor stubbornly refused to eat the food that someone else had prepared.

'Well,' she exclaimed indignantly, 'I don't want to eat that stuff – it's not my thing at all! They keep bringing it and I don't know why – I've never asked them. At least Billy likes it. He loves it actually. Especially the beef and Yorkshire puddings!'

The rich meals-on-wheels food had a tendency to give Billy an upset tummy, which was one of the reasons I had to see him so often. An added complication was that the soft faeces would get stuck to the fur around his bottom. My job, every few months, was to trim away the matted fur. Not particularly pleasant, but actually very satisfying. A quick whizz with the clippers brought about an almost instant cure. The most instant cure of all though, was the removal on one occasion of a boiled sweet. The sweet had stuck so closely to the little dog's fur that everyone initially thought it was an aggressive and sinister tumour. But, when I got up close to inspect the mass, I noticed a minty smell. It was a Fox's Glacier Mint. No radical surgery was required, just some deft action with scissors!

Anyway, Mrs Taylor was always grateful for my help, both in caring for her dogs and for helping her in her dotage. I once called to see Billy and ended up retuning her TV.

'All I can get is this thing called Al Jazeera and it's not really what I want,' she sighed when I asked her what she was watching. I offered to try to sort it out, which resulted in a diagnostic process more involved than for any canine illness.

After another visit some weeks later, as I was about to leave, Mrs Taylor explained that she had been clearing out some of her stuff and asked whether I would like anything. She was very insistent and it seemed rude to decline, so I found myself leaving with a portrait, in oil paint on canvas, of her little poodle and a porcelain figurine of a barn owl. Grateful as I was, I doubted that either would make it to my mantelpiece!

One of her eclectic gifts, however, is still very much on display. It is another porcelain figure, but this time in the rather unlikely shape of a bulldog. Even more unlikely is that this stoic symbol of all things British has a burgundy lampshade on its head. I had called in to visit a lovely couple, Mr and Mrs T., whose beloved bulldog, Elsie, had just died. It was a sad occasion. I had seen a lot of her as she had become more and more poorly and had got to know both her and her owners well. As we reminisced about Elsie and her funny ways, I commented on the rather magnificent lamp.

'Well Julian, if it reminds you of our Elsie, you must have it!' exclaimed Mrs T. And so there it sits, proudly and resolutely, on my kitchen table and, more than six months later, it still makes me smile and reminds me of the lovely patient of which it is the reincarnation.

The list of similar gifts is long: a smorgasbord of merchandise from the Isle of Man, including keyrings, cheeses, tea towels and mugs from a fan of *The Yorkshire Vet* who lives there; a generous bottle of champagne from a couple who I knew could certainly not afford such a luxury – again given after I had delivered the final injection to provide a peaceful end to a precious life; a rug made from the fleece of an alpaca, which arrived from a lady who lived in London. She was moving house and needed to find a new home for the rug, which she had brought back from South America some fifty years before. I had never met this lady, but she had seen me on TV and knew I had an interest in alpacas. It was touching that she had identified me as a suitable keeper and had gone to the trouble of packaging the well-travelled rug and posting it all the way to North Yorkshire.

And then there was the man who arrived outside the practice on a moped. Without removing his motorcycle helmet, and with very few words, he delivered a book for me. The book was entitled *Diseases of Canaries* and was written by the Birdman of Alcatraz. I was out on calls so, sadly, I couldn't thank him personally. To this day, nobody knows where he came from. Could he *actually* have brought the book from Alcatraz?

But, of all these gifts, Duffy's wine was certainly the most useful of all. When I returned to see Nick at the wine shop, he was still confused.

'I've been investigating and it's intriguing,' he explained. 'There's none of your wine to be found anywhere, I'm afraid. But what I do know is that the wine grown next door, just over the wall, is *the most expensive wine in the world!*'

Then he added, 'That's not yours though, because yours isn't as good as that . . . The closest I can find is one called . . .' At this point I drifted off – much as I was fascinated by my special bottle, I knew this was not a genre with which I wanted to become superfamiliar – but I re-engaged just moments later: '. . . and it costs just over eight hundred pounds a bottle.'

Had I been tasting my next-level-up Burgundy, I would surely have spat it all over the floor, but I wasn't, so I didn't. 'Wow,' was all I could say. It suddenly seemed a long time since the bags of potatoes and armfuls of swedes of my early days as a vet. I wondered where I could find a partridge or a guinea fowl to cook to have with my wine later that evening.

'I'll lend you my Burgundy glass,' Nick added. 'To appreciate this fully you need the right food, but you also need the right glass. It's handmade and it will allow you to enjoy it properly.'

The following Saturday night, with Nick's enormous glass in my hand, I made plans for the grand opening. Anne was going to have just a glass, not being a fan of red wine, so most of it had my name on it. In the end I didn't have a partridge, or any guinea fowl, and the most expensive bottle of wine that I will ever see, hold and taste was consumed, with great appreciation, alongside nothing more fancy than a chorizo-topped pizza. I have to say, it was utterly exquisite. I raised an oversized glass to Duffy, the little Westie with the oversized waist and an almost inoperable, oversized liver tumour.

'Thank you for the wine, Duffy, but more importantly, thank you for making it through the operation,' I toasted. The bottle of wine was fantastic, but the satisfaction of saving this little dog's life would linger long after the cherry and liquorice notes had left my palate. I like drinking lovely wine, but what I really love is saving the lives of little dogs and making their owners very, very happy.

22. Lambing with the Family

Ten thirty at night is not the worst time to get a call to lamb a sheep. The worst time is when you have been in bed for a couple of hours and have descended into a deep sleep, only to be wrenched back out of it by the phone. You lie there in complete confusion, trying to work out what is real and what isn't as you haul yourself back into consciousness. So, while I would not be getting an early night on this cold February evening, at least my sleep had not been disturbed. Not yet anyway!

Jenny, one of the nurses, was taking the emergency phone calls for the night. She gave me the name and number of the farmer and a brief summary of the problem, which I noted on the chaotic-looking scrap of paper next to the phone. It was covered with scribbled names, phone numbers and descriptions of various animal ailments. I am always reluctant to throw these pieces of paper away, in case I need to find a name or number again – I should really keep a notebook for the purpose, but I never get around to being that organised. Anyway, I squeezed the number onto an empty corner and made the call to discuss the sheep.

'Well, I just don't know what to mek on it,' explained the farmer, whose name was Ben. He had a distinctive broad Yorkshire accent, which immediately threw me. I knew this Ben was a goat farmer and yet he was speaking of a problem with a sheep. I had presumed it was a different Ben, another farmer I knew well, who had a similar-sounding surname but a different accent.

'And it's a sheep and not a goat?' I asked, trying to reassure myself that I had the right farmer.

'Aye, I've got abart fifty or so. They're me dad's really, but I'm looking after 'em this year. He's not so good now.' That explained it.

'Any 'ow, this ewe, well, I can't mek nowt of her. She's on lambing, definite, but it just feels all wrong to me. I've never felt owt like it. I feel a complete plonker, calling you out on a night like tonight, yer know, for a commercial yow and all, but I just don't know what else to do.'

I knew Ben well. His voice was as unmistakable as the rest of him. The best way to describe him was as a Yorkshire version of the comedian Peter Kay. I first met him at a dinner event for the Young Famers' group of which he was part, some months before I moved to work at the surgery in Boroughbridge. Ben was part of the glue that held Farnley Estates Young Farmers' Club together. He was a dynamic, whirling dervish of energy and enthusiasm, one of the characters who helped the club to thrive. I had been asked, following a chance meeting with the club secretary at a bookshop in Scarborough, to do an after-dinner speech at their event, whose aim was to raise funds for a couple of local charities. One of those charities was a fantastic organisation called Candlelighters, which helps children and their families suffering with cancer in and around Yorkshire. I was more than happy to contribute. Ben was the compère for the evening, which was held in the village hall in picturesque Darley, on the cusp of the hills between Nidderdale and Wharfedale. He captivated the room with his charisma and I feared that, having to follow his superb comic work on the microphone, I would be a rather disappointing act.

We sat next to each other during dinner and covered pretty much all topics relating to farming, over the pie and peas. As I watched the pints of Black Sheep bitter slip down one after another, I offered Ben a lift home at the end of the night – I would be driving right past his farm on my way back to Thirsk.

'I'll be raight, Julian, but thank you.' He nodded. 'I'll call it a day after this one, I think. I've got Jacob here too.' He pointed towards his youngest son, who was chatting with a circle of mates in one corner of the large village hall. 'He's got school tomorrow, so I'll not be having a late one.'

After the meal, I got to my feet, took Ben's microphone and spoke about my recent experiences as a vet, an author and also being on the telly. I am not naturally comfortable doing this sort of thing but the audience, which consisted of farmers of all ages and plenty of young kids, seemed fascinated. Whichever way you look at it, my life has taken an interesting turn. The questions continued after I'd finished speaking and the pints kept flowing for Ben and for many others. Sometime after midnight, people started to disperse, the chairs were stacked and the room tidied.

'Julian, thank you very much. That was magic,' Ben effused, before going on to add, 'any chance of that lift home?'

Once I had arrived at the Boroughbridge practice, I started to see Ben regularly in my professional capacity. His main farming enterprise was a herd of dairy goats – an unusual niche but one that Ben and his family loved. 'I just luv goats,' I have heard him declare on many occasions.

During his busiest time of year, when the goats were kidding,

Ben would call us in regularly to disbud the little kids. Goats' horns are particularly troublesome, causing injury to one another as well as getting damaged. I remember, early in my veterinary career, the demise of my favourite shirt as a result of a belligerent billy goat's horn; it tore a huge, irreparable hole in the chest area, luckily just missing my skin.

Not all goat farmers would go to the lengths of disbudding (that is, removing the rubbery buds of horns not yet grown) all their baby kids. The procedure has to be done under general anaesthetic as goats cannot tolerate local anaesthetic in the way calves can. This means time and money, but Ben wanted to do things properly. A busy morning would see sixty week-old kids having their little horn buds removed, in a makeshift operating theatre on the farm. He had developed a superbly slick system that made for very pleasant work. It was efficient and effective and it was rewarding to see one baby goat after another recover from its deep slumbers, wobble to its feet in the golden straw and, within just minutes, start jumping and skipping as if nothing had happened.

'Look at 'em laking around,' said Ben, hands on hips as he stood back and admired his kids, just as if they were his actual kids. 'I could watch 'em all day.' (Laking is a Yorkshire term for playing, not often heard but very evocative.)

The goats seldom had any problems, so other than to do the horn job, I didn't visit the farm very often. Ben was very experienced at delivering both lambs and goat kids, but this evening's case was clearly causing even him confusion. My summation from the phone conversation was that the ewe had a uterine torsion. This is a fairly common condition in cattle, but is rare in sheep. The whole uterus twists along its axis, rendering the birth canal completely obstructed. The usual assessment from a farmer is exactly as Ben had described: 'It just feels completely wrong – I can't mek nowt of it!'

When I got there, Ben and his two young sons, Jacob and Charlie, greeted me. From my first evening in Darley with Ben, I knew the boys were both committed young farmers. They had been allowed to stay up late to watch this peculiar lambing. It was February half-term, so there was no school to get to the next morning, and watching a vet deliver lambs was clearly far more interesting than boring old bed.

The only course of action when the uterus is twisted is to deliver the lambs via Caesarean section, so there would be plenty of excitement for Jacob and Charlie. I applied lubricant and carefully felt inside. My hand slid in easily to my wrist, but then would go no further. There was the telltale sign of a blind-ending vagina, which means it is, just like a sock with its toe end tied into a knot.

I explained the situation to Ben.

'It's impossible to correct the twist in a ewe without doing a Caesarean section.'

Then to the boys, 'Can you get me a couple of buckets of warm water please lads?'

Both young faces lit up with excitement and they scuttled off into the darkness. Ben hadn't seen a Caesarean section performed on a sheep before – and neither had his lads – so I talked him through the process.

I learnt my sheep Caesarean method while working in the north of Scotland, in Thurso, just a stone's throw from John o'Groats. It is a wild and beautiful part of the world and one that is full of sheep. On a busy day in spring, there could be a queue of five or more Land Rovers with trailers attached, each with an expectant mother inside. The lambing shed at the surgery was just like a maternity ward and the process became something of a production line.

The standard surgical technique, favoured by vet schools

219

teaching students the tools of their trade, involves making a long vertical surgical incision in the left flank of the sheep as it lies on its right side. This part of the ewe is covered in fleece and under the skin are three layers of muscle, each of which needs to be incised. However, the technique I learnt from those amazing vets in Scotland involved a smaller incision under the left flank, just above the udder and in a horizontal direction. There is just one layer of muscle to cut through and the uterus is directly under the incision. The process, in capable hands, takes about ten minutes, and is much quicker than the standard approach. When opening up an abdomen in a non-sterile farm environment, time is of the essence. The more quickly the surgical site is closed, the better, so quick, efficient surgery always comes up trumps. Ben had seen neither technique, so even though I was at pains to explain the process, he wasn't really concerned about where I made my incision, so long as his ewe and her lambs were safe and sound.

Jacob and Charlie had returned by now, each with a bucket brimming with warm water. Both boys were also brimming with excitement and they bobbed up and down outside the sheep pen as they waited to see what was in store for them and the sheep.

I have done this operation hundreds of time but it still gives me a thrill. There is jeopardy at every stage: Will the ewe lie still? Will the lambs be alive? Will it go according to plan?

Even though it is a routine procedure, there is nothing routine about bringing new life into the world, and I was excited too. I knew Jacob and Charlie would be transfixed and I hoped, as much for their sakes as that of the sheep and her as yet unborn lambs, that tonight would be a success.

Everything progressed nicely. The patient was well behaved as Ben held her. I'm not sure if he was actually murmuring words of calming encouragement in her ear, but it certainly looked as if he was. He occasionally offered positive comments in my direction: 'By, that's nifty, Julian! I can't believe you're right inside her stomach!'

His sons stood, open-mouthed and motionless, absorbing every part of the operation.

With all these onlookers hanging on every cut of my scalpel and every suture I placed, I could easily have wilted under the pressure, but it went as smoothly as I could have hoped. First one, then a second lamb emerged into the cold February night air. Ben kept a firm hold on the ewe while I started to sew everything back together. Jacob and Charlie took over the duties of lamb resuscitation. It was literally all hands on deck and I was glad of the help of these two budding young farmers.

The first few moments after delivery give a fairly reliable indication of the viability of the lamb, and I glanced over to see how they were doing. There was a small gasp and then a brief muscular spasm from each one, as the boys continued to rub them vigorously to remove fluid and mucus from their airways, exposed to air for the first time. They both knew exactly what to do, but I sensed all was not going to plan. There were a couple more spasms from each lamb, but from my position beside the ewe, I couldn't tell whether they were proper breaths or reflex, agonal gasps as the lambs tried to cling to their nascent life. Agonal gasps are the final gasps at an attempt to salvage life. Usually a reflex, after meaningful life has finished, these terminal gasps can give the illusion that life is still there and that there is still hope. Vets and experienced farmers know this is not the case. Agonal gasps are false hope of life. I was busy with the ewe and her uterus, anxious to get a good and quick seal to the incisions I'd made, and Ben was occupied holding the patient, so it was down to the lads. In a few frenetic minutes, it was finished and the ewe was back together; but the two lambs were not sitting up, spluttering and flapping their ears as we had all hoped and expected. Jacob and Charlie had done their best, but the lambs were not quite right and never properly came to life. Were they early, were they late, should I have been quicker with my surgery? We'll never know.

Ben put a hand on the shoulder of each of his sons.

'You did your best, lads. It just wasn't to be tonight. At least the ewe's okay – I'll maybe try and foster that spare lamb onto her later. Anyway, it's bedtime now and it's late.'

The words of encouragement and consolation did not do much to lift the boys' spirits, but they were farmer's sons and they knew that things did not always end well. Despite the sadness of this evening, they both knew there would be happy endings to come during the lambing time ahead.

Lambing time is busy for farmers and, consequently, vets too. Most nights during February and March are disturbed and both vets and farmers get more and more weary. However, after a late night with Ben and his family during my night on call in the week, I was really hoping for a quiet weekend. It was something of an unrealistic ambition. I was just retrieving my casserole from the oven one Sunday evening, after a non-stop day, when the phone went again. I groaned. I was hungry and the casserole smelt delicious. But, there was another lambing and it was miles away – right up in the Dales in a little village called Grantley. The farmer's daughter sounded anxious as she relayed the problem: 'My mum and dad are up there now with the sheep. It's not at our usual farm, because we're having some building work done at home, so the sheep are at a neighbour's until it's finished. It's a bit of a trek but it should be okay. Dad says he'll meet you at the end of the lane. The snow is coming down up here, but you'll be all right if you have a 4x4.'

My heart sank. Not only would it be a long journey, a long night and a late tea, but there was also a chance I could get stuck in the snow. There was wind and rain in Thirsk and it was certainly cold, but until I'd had this weather update from the Dales, it hadn't occurred to me that there might be snow higher up.

When my veterinary work was based around Thirsk and the Hambleton Hills, a call up to Sutton Bank in winter or early spring would often mean a change in the weather. It was always a few degrees colder up there, with a prevailing wind from the east, which could mean snow drifts a metre deep across the drover's road along the top of the escarpment or the roads on to Helmsley and the rest of Ryedale while down in the Vale of York there was only rain or sleet. As I thought about it, I realised that Grantley must be at a similar altitude – on the drive back across Nidderdale from Pateley Bridge on my way home to Thirsk, I am always in awe of the expansive view of the White Horse of Kilburn with the setting sun reflecting off Whitestonecliffe, and it feels as if you are looking across at it from a similar elevation.

This evening, I wound my way upwards and round narrow, twisting lanes flanked by drystone walls – some immaculate and some collapsing – and the rain gradually changed to sleet, making a different pattern on the windscreen. Before long, the sleet changed to snow and the dark roads and walls wore a blanket of white.

I had another problem as well as the weather. I didn't know exactly where I was going. There are no streetlights in these remote parts of Yorkshire, so it was completely dark, and the satnav was notoriously unreliable on these country lanes. I had scribbled down some directions on my trusty bit of paper, and then I'd written them out again, more clearly so I could read them properly (my handwriting is terrible). I just had to hope I had written everything down accurately. Missing just one of the crucial turns would render the rest of the chain of instructions completely useless, so I crossed my fingers as I pressed on into the gloom. At least my trusty Subaru would not let me down in these challenging conditions.

After what seemed like ages, I came upon a car parked in the darkness by the side of the road, with its hazard warning lights flashing. As I approached, its headlights flashed, lighting up the road in front of it. I paused, unsure what to make of this, as the car set off slowly into the middle of nowhere. Hoping that this was, in fact, the farmer kindly come out onto the lane to guide me in on this horrible night and not some psychotic murderer who was luring this gullible and unsuspecting traveller to his death, I followed the car across an open moor, up and up, to a place where the stone walls disappeared. Then we turned right, down an even narrower lane, before the vehicle came to a halt, its lights went out and everything went dark. I'd read about this sort of thing in books!

Thankfully, a cheerful face appeared at my car window.

'Well done! You've made it, thank you for coming. What a night to be out! This snow just keeps on coming! Anyhow, it's this ewe: we're having a problem and we need some help and you're the man for the job. Everything is harder with our sheep up here. It is a sod of a place to find, even in the daytime!'

I was confident by now that this was definitely a sheep farmer and not a murderer, so I pulled on my wellies, grabbed a bottle of lube and followed him into the dim barn. At least if he did still turn out to be a murderer, I could lather him with lubricant and make my escape. But he didn't. Instead, he introduced me to his wife, who was swaddled in layers of scarves and hats and was just as pleased to see me. She was kneeling, deep in straw, with a sheep who was clearly struggling. The wind howled and whistled and spindrift squirted snowflakes through the slits in

224

the Yorkshire boards that made up the lambing shed. I knelt down to be closer to the sheep. Down at her level, it was remarkably snug, sheltered and warm; it would be a pleasant place to get to work and also, if all went to plan, a nice place for a newborn lamb.

The couple quickly introduced themselves as Mr and Mrs Robinson and explained everything about the Texel who was in difficulty.

'We just can't get it out,' was the final summary of the lambing situation. I cleaned my arms in the bucket of ice-cold antiseptic solution and applied a generous amount of lubricant to my hand and lower arm, before making a gentle exploration inside the ewe's vagina. This is always exciting, as it is the point at which I can make my first assessment of the lamb, its presentation and the likelihood of delivering it successfully. On an evening like this, the sudden sensation of warmth from the internal body temperature of the sheep is hard to describe. It is almost like a burning feeling. It's a nice feeling, though, and I reached further inside to get the hang of the problem.

'What's it like? Do you think you'll be able to get it out, Julian? We are so worried. It's our best sheep.'

Mrs Robinson talked constantly, keen for details. She need not have worried, because I always try to provide a running commentary of what I am doing, with both lambings and calvings. The farmer is always anxious, but has absolutely no clue of my progress unless I tell them what I can feel. It seems rude not to explain.

The lamb was large (Texels often are) and there was a leg back. Lambs need to be born, under most circumstances, with both front legs pointing forward and the head lying in between. There simply isn't sufficient space to get most lambs out if one leg is bent backward. With some careful manipulation, I managed to flick up the leg in question and extend the elbow. Mrs Robinson's level of excitement was rising with each step of the process. I finally applied traction to both legs together and eased the skin of the ewe's vulva around the crown of the emerging forehead. The rest of the lamb slid out easily and there was a similar outpouring of emotion from the farmers.

'Oh Julian, you are an absolute *angel*! I'm so pleased. You are so clever and you made it look easy!'

I think it was the most emotional thanks I've ever had from a grateful farmer. I'd certainly never been called an angel before!

As the three of us watched the lamb, slimy but healthy, shake its head, flap its ears and make a bid for the teat, we continued our conversation with much more relief.

A former colleague always used to advise me: 'Never make it look easy! A farmer won't pay if he doesn't think you've earned your corn, so huff and puff a bit and, if necessary, keep it in for a bit longer!'

This has never been a philosophy to which I've subscribed; I don't think deception has any part in veterinary practice. I had a long journey home, through deep snow. I had no reason to linger on the farm for longer than I needed to on this freezing cold and wintery night. And what's more, my casserole was still waiting for me!

Acknowledgements

I'll try to keep this brief. First thanks must go to Alan McCormack, my boss at Rae, Bean and Partners, Boroughbridge, for allowing me into his family of vets and staff. You really didn't know what you were letting yourself in for when we talked about me coming to work with you and your practice – I hope it's been worth it, that it's been a fun and a happy time having me there.

Alistair Rae, who came to see me on my very first day, wishing me all the best in my new job at his old practice: thank you for your support from day one; and also Georgina Bean, wife of the late Vic Bean. Vic's ethos lives on in the practice and exudes from every corner. I hope I've followed in his footsteps to some extent and I hope he would have been pleased to have had me practising in Boroughbridge.

David Riding, my literary agent, is someone to whom I owe huge thanks and gratitude. I suspect I've not been his easiest client (I'm sorry – I'm new to the world of books, I'm just a vet after all), but you've helped me hugely, with support, encouragement where necessary and freedom and flexibility where appropriate. As you know, this book would not have been here without your help.

Paul Stead and his team at Daisybeck Studios – thank you. What an adventure it's been!

Fiona Rose, Hannah Black and all the fantastic staff at Hodder and Stoughton, thank you. This book represents my first foray into the 'proper' book world. I hope I've done you justice!

Anne, once again, thank you for helping, editing, removing unnecessary punctuation and for supporting my madcap stuff. It does get a bit easier, doesn't it?

I must thank the animal owners who feature in this book. Some are under pseudonyms, to protect identity and client confidentiality; some are under their real names and the real names of their cats, dogs and other creatures both great and small. And especially Christine. Your beloved Sid finally gets into a book! Without farmers, the pet-owning public and your animals, this book would not exist and my life as a vet would be very different.

And finally, thanks go to you, the reader, chugging through this final section of my fifth book. I hope you've enjoyed it and that my account of moving practices has been uplifting and positive, rather than negative and gloomy. It has been a challenging period in my life and it has not been easy, moving practices and writing about it, but both have confirmed my belief that a person *has* to do the right thing. Sticking to your principles is the right thing to do, no matter how hard it is and how big the challenges are. Do that and you'll not go far wrong. That's what I say anyway.